Psychological and Cognitive Impact
of Critical Illness

Psychological and Cognitive Impact of Critical Illness

EDITED BY

O. JOSEPH BIENVENU, MD, PHD

Associate Professor, Psychiatry and Behavioral Sciences
Director, General Hospital Psychiatry Inpatient Consultation Service
Johns Hopkins Hospital
Co-Director, Johns Hopkins Anxiety Disorders Clinic
and Residents' Outpatient Continuity Clinic
Johns Hopkins University School of Medicine

CHRISTINA JONES, RN, PHD

Nurse Consultant
Critical Care Rehabilitation
Whiston Hospital

RAMONA O. HOPKINS, PHD

Professor, Psychology and Neuroscience
Director, Neuroscience Center
Brigham Young University
Clinical Research Investigator, Pulmonary and Critical Care Division
Department of Medicine
Intermountain Medical Center
Center for Humanizing Critical Care
Intermountain Healthcare

OXFORD
UNIVERSITY PRESS

OXFORD
UNIVERSITY PRESS

Oxford University Press is a department of the University of Oxford. It furthers
the University's objective of excellence in research, scholarship, and education
by publishing worldwide. Oxford is a registered trade mark of Oxford University
Press in the UK and certain other countries.

Published in the United States of America by Oxford University Press
198 Madison Avenue, New York, NY 10016, United States of America.

CIP data is on file at the Library of Congress
ISBN 978-0-19-939869-0

9 8 7 6 5 4 3 2 1

Printed by Webcom, Inc., Canada

This material is not intended to be, and should not be considered, a substitute for medical or other
professional advice. Treatment for the conditions described in this material is highly dependent on
the individual circumstances. And, while this material is designed to offer accurate information with
respect to the subject matter covered and to be current as of the time it was written, research and
knowledge about medical and health issues is constantly evolving and dose schedules for medications
are being revised continually, with new side effects recognized and accounted for regularly. Readers
must therefore always check the product information and clinical procedures with the most up-to-date
published product information and data sheets provided by the manufacturers and the most recent
codes of conduct and safety regulation. The publisher and the authors make no representations or
warranties to readers, express or implied, as to the accuracy or completeness of this material. Without
limiting the foregoing, the publisher and the authors make no representations or warranties as to the
accuracy or efficacy of the drug dosages mentioned in the material. The authors and the publisher do
not accept, and expressly disclaim, any responsibility for any liability, loss or risk that may be claimed
or incurred as a consequence of the use and/ or application of any of the contents of this material.

CONTENTS

CONTRIBUTORS   VII

OVERVIEW: PSYCHOLOGICAL AND COGNITIVE IMPACT
OF CRITICAL ILLNESS   XI
O. Joseph Bienvenu, Christina Jones, and Ramona O. Hopkins

1. Testimonies in Understanding the Psychological and Cognitive
   Problems Faced by Survivors of Critical Illness   1
   Christina Jones, Peter Gibb, and Ramona O. Hopkins

2. Delirium in Critically Ill Patients   31
   Mark van den Boogaard and Paul Rood

3. Critical Illness and Long-Term Cognitive Impairment   47
   Ramona O. Hopkins, Maria E. Carlo, and James C. Jackson

4. Psychological Impact of Critical Illness   69
   O. Joseph Bienvenu and Christina Jones

5. Rehabilitation Psychology Insights for Treatment of Critical Illness
   Survivors   105
   Jennifer E. Jutte, James C. Jackson, and Ramona O. Hopkins

6. Prevention and Treatment of Posttraumatic Stress and Depressive
   Phenomena in Critical Illness Survivors   141
   Christina Jones and O. Joseph Bienvenu

7. Supporting Pediatric Patients and Their Families during and after
   Intensive Care Treatment   169
   Gillian Colville

8. Family Response to Critical Illness   191
   Judy E. Davidson and Giora Netzer

INDEX   211

O. Joseph Bienvenu, MD, PhD
Associate Professor, Psychiatry and
    Behavioral Sciences
Director, General Hospital Psychiatry
    Inpatient Consultation Service
Johns Hopkins Hospital
Co-Director, Johns Hopkins Anxiety
    Disorders Clinic and Residents'
    Outpatient Continuity Clinic
Johns Hopkins University School
    of Medicine
Baltimore, Maryland

Mark van den Boogaard, PhD
Critical Care Nurse, Nursing
    Scientist
Research Intensive Care Unit
Radboud University
    Medical Centre
Nijmegen, Gelderland, the
    Netherlands

Maria E. Carlo, MD
Center for Health Services
    Research, Department of
    Medicine
Divisions of Geriatric Medicine
    and General Internal Medicine
    and Public Health
Vanderbilt University School of
    Medicine
Nashville, Tennessee

**Gillian Colville, BSc,
    MPhil, AFBPsS**
Consultant Clinical
    Psychologist
Paediatric Psychology Service
St. George's University
    Hospitals NHS
    Foundation Trust
London, England

**Judy E. Davidson DNP,
  RN, FCCM**
Evidence Based Practice and
  Research Nurse Liaison
Case Western Reserve University
University of California–San
  Diego
San Diego, California

Peter Gibb
Chief Executive, ICUsteps
Milton Keynes, Buckinghamshire,
  England

Ramona O. Hopkins, PhD
Professor, Psychology and
  Neuroscience
Director, Neuroscience
  Center
Brigham Young University
Provo, Utah
Clinical Research Investigator,
  Pulmonary and Critical Care
  Division
Department of Medicine
Intermountain Medical Center
Center for Humanizing
  Critical Care
Intermountain Health Care
Murray, Utah

James C. Jackson, PsyD
Center for Health Services Research
Department of Medicine
Department of Psychiatry
ICU Recovery Center
Division of Allergy, Pulmonary,
  and Critical Care Medicine
Divisions of Geriatric Medicine
  and General Internal Medicine
  and Public Health
Vanderbilt University School of
  Medicine
Research Service, Department of
  Veterans Affairs Medical Center
Tennessee Valley Healthcare System
Nashville, Tennessee

Christina Jones, PhD
Nurse Consultant
Critical Care Rehabilitation
Whiston Hospital
Liverpool, Merseyside, England

Jennifer E. Jutte, MPH, PhD
Department of Rehabilitation
  Medicine
University of Washington School
  of Medicine
Harborview Medical Center
Seattle, Washington

Giora Netzer, MD, MSCE
Associate Professor
Medicine, Epidemiology &
    Public Health
University of Maryland School of
    Medicine
Baltimore, Maryland

Paul Rood, BSc
Critical Care Nurse, PhD
    Candidate
Research Intensive Care Unit
Radboud University Medical Centre
Nijmegen, Gelderland, the
    Netherlands

OVERVIEW: PSYCHOLOGICAL AND COGNITIVE
IMPACT OF CRITICAL ILLNESS

Millions of patients are treated in intensive care units (ICUs) each year; notably, more than a million elderly patients survive critical illness yearly in the United States alone.[1] The number of survivors is growing as a result of advances in critical care medicine and decreasing mortality rates.[2] Unfortunately, many critical illness survivors have substantial morbidity.[3] Physical, psychological, and cognitive impairments are particularly common—so much so that a group of us coined the term *post-intensive care syndrome* (or PICS) to help raise awareness.[4,5]

Patients surviving critical illnesses are often quite weak. The causes include muscle disuse due to immobility, as well as nerve and muscle damage due to systemic inflammation and organ dysfunction. Physical therapy, hopefully begun in the ICU, is vital.[4] But weakness is only one of the problems critical illness survivors and their loved ones face. Unfortunately, many survivors are left with cognitive impairment (e.g., impaired memory, attention, and executive functioning), as well as distress-related psychiatric phenomena like posttraumatic stress and depression.[4]

In order to understand what it is like to be (or have been) critically ill, it is useful to imagine oneself in a hospital bed surrounded by machines that emit lights and noises of various sorts. One often will have a tube down one's throat connected to a breathing machine, and nurses come in intermittently to perform painful (and life-saving) suctioning of secretions. One will typically be connected to a number of tubes, including central intravenous lines, arterial lines, urinary catheters, and others. Inserting these tubes will have been painful, and if one has lost one's cognitive faculties as a result of failing organs and/or sedative medications, any of these procedures can seem like purposeful torture. To top it off, one is relatively helpless and unable to communicate easily. In sum, being critically ill and requiring intensive care is *stressful*—to one's organs (including the brain) and to one's self.

In the following chapters, we and our colleagues outline what we know about neuropsychiatric problems in critical illness survivors, including what we might do to prevent long-term impairment. Chapter 1 provides a historical overview by early researchers and advocates in this field. Chapter 2 sets the stage with a discussion of delirium in critically ill patients—a very common neuropsychiatric problem *in the midst of* critical illness. Chapters 3 and 4 discuss the nature and epidemiology of long-term cognitive impairment and emotional distress-related psychiatric problems, respectively, in critical illness survivors. Chapters 5 and 6 discuss prevention and early intervention efforts, which are still being developed and tested. Chapters 7 and 8 focus on children with critical illness, as well as the families of critically ill patients.

In writing this book, we were motivated by powerful experiences with many critical illness survivors and their loved ones. We hope that it is instructive, but we also hope that readers will join us in developing better, collaborative approaches to improve the lives of our patients.

REFERENCES

1. Wunsch H, Guerra C, Barnato AE, Angus DC, Li G, Linde-Zwirble WT. Three-year outcomes for Medicare beneficiaries who survive intensive care. *JAMA.* 2010;303(9):849–856.
2. Prescott HC, Kepreos KM, Wiitala WL, Iwashyna TJ. Temporal changes in the influence of hospitals and regional healthcare networks on severe sepsis mortality. *Crit Care Med.* 2015;43(7):1368–1374.

3. Iwashyna TJ. Survivorship will be the defining challenge of critical care in the 21st century. *Ann Intern Med*. 2010;153(3):204–205.

4. Needham DM, Davidson J, Cohen H, et al. Improving long-term outcomes after discharge from intensive care unit: report from a stakeholders' conference. *Crit Care Med*. 2012;40(2):502–509.

5. Elliott D, Davidson JE, Harvey MA, et al. Exploring the scope of post-intensive care syndrome therapy and care: engagement of non-critical care providers and survivors in a second stakeholders meeting. *Crit Care Med*. 2014;42(12):2518–2526.

Testimonies in Understanding the Psychological and Cognitive Problems Faced by Survivors of Critical Illness

CHRISTINA JONES, PETER GIBB, AND RAMONA O. HOPKINS

THE INTENSIVE CARE UNIT (ICU) NURSE TURNED RESEARCHER—CHRISTINA JONES

Severe illness as a cause of fragmentary memory and amnesia

When I did my nursing degree I did an arts option of ancient history for a year. I discovered that nightmares and hallucinations had long been reported to accompany febrile illness, particularly before the advent of antibiotics. As far back as the first century A.D., Celsus described delirium and observed that it was a sign that a fever was severe. He regarded delirium as a form of insanity:[1]

[I]nsanity is really there when a continuous dementia begins, when the patient, although up till then in his senses, yet entertains certain vain imaginings; the insanity becomes established when the mind becomes at the mercy of such imaginings. (Celsus 3.18. 1–3)

Celsus also recorded that this delirium had been described by the Greeks. Somehow we had forgotten this.

ICU PSYCHOSIS

In the 1980s the term *ICU psychosis* began to be used as a catch-all phrase to explain patient agitation in critical care. It was defined as an "acute organic brain syndrome involving impaired intellectual functioning which occurs in patients who are being treated within a critical care unit. When the impairment is of such magnitude that the patient cannot adequately judge reality, the syndrome can be termed an ICU psychosis."[2] Hallucinations, sleep disorders, and confusion were all widely reported, and a link was suggested between the ICU environment and psychiatric disturbance.[3] In the literature the term *ICU psychosis* has now been largely replaced by the more precise term *delirium*; the link to the ICU environment was a misinterpretation of the impact of severe illness and sedative and opioid medication in precipitating delirium. As patients who are critically ill and admitted to ICU are so seriously ill, it is not surprising that delirium should be so common in that setting.

Psychological impact of critical illness

Despite the literature about "ICU psychosis" and the reporting of hallucinations and nightmares experienced by patients in the ICU in the 1980s, there appeared to be little understanding of the long-term effects of critical illness. At the end of the 1980s, in the United Kingdom, a chance conversation between two ICU consultants led to a follow-up study in which patients were called back to a dedicated ICU outpatient clinic. The ICU at Whiston Hospital had a long tradition of medical physicians being involved in patient care, and one of those physicians, Dr. Steve Atherton, was seeing recovering ICU patients in his normal medical respiratory clinics. He noticed that they seemed to take a long time to recover, and he discussed this with another ICU consultant, Dr. Richard Griffiths, who was a physician with an interest in muscle physiology. Research funding was found in order to employ a research nurse—me—to set up the outpatient clinic in June 1990. In talking with patients and their families in the clinic 2, 6, and sometimes 12 months after ICU discharge, it became clear that many patients were unable to recall the period of critical illness.[4] This lack of memory for the period of critical illness made it difficult for patients to understand why their recovery was so slow.[5] Patients felt that the recovery phase of their critical illness was the most stressful period as they learned how ill and close to death they had been.[6] In an early follow-up study at Whiston Hospital using questionnaires to examine health-related quality of life, 41% of patients had reduced their social activities and 25% reported being irritable with their family members at 6 months post-ICU.[4] Twenty-five percent of longer-stay patients (≥5 days) scored highly for anxiety and depression at 2 months post-ICU. Despite reporting amnesia for their time in ICU, many patients reported recalling vivid memories of nightmares and hallucinations, which they found difficult to separate from reality.[7] For some patients their only memories of the ICU were nightmares, often of a persecutory nature or involving being subjected to torture.[4] A number of patients reported a Capgras-type delusion, with ICU staff or their family being replaced by aliens or waxwork or shop dummies (see Case History 1).[8] This sort of delusion was first reported in 1923, as "l'illusion des sosies," by Capgras and Reboul-Lachaux,[9] in a case report of a 53-year-old woman who believed her husband and children had been replaced by doubles. In Capgras syndrome, the doubles are normally of close family or friends, and patients frequently report that the doubles are evil or dangerous. In addition, patients are often paranoid and may suffer from feelings of depersonalization.

CASE HISTORY 1: CAPGRAS DELUSION IN THE ICU

A 42-year-old woman was admitted to the ICU in respiratory failure, having developed pneumonia and the adult respiratory distress syndrome following extensive surgery for a squamous cell carcinoma, secondary to Crohn's disease. During her ICU stay she was ventilated for the first 5 days, followed by 5 days of spontaneous respiration through a tracheostomy tube. During the second 5 days, when she was being weaned from the ventilator, nursing staff thought that she looked terrified, and for the final 3 days she was not able to sleep. At the end of the weaning period, her tracheostomy was removed and she was able to speak. She confided to the nurse caring for her that she was very frightened about something and wanted to talk to someone about the memories she had of her illness. I was asked to see her and she confided to me that her memories of the previous 3 days were of all her family, with the exception of her mother, being replaced by aliens. She recognized the faces of her family members but knew somehow that they were, in fact, aliens. She had been terrified of going to sleep because she had been convinced that the aliens were waiting for the opportunity to take over her body. At the time of our interview she did realize that this experience had been a delusion, but she was frightened that it showed she was going mad and that it might happen again. Once discharged to the general wards, I followed up with her, and she remained distressed by her memories. When she was subsequently told, 2 weeks after ICU discharge, that she would need further plastic surgery to cover a large skin defect, she initially refused. Further discussion revealed that she was frightened of a recurrence of the delusion following a general anesthetic. The anesthetist involved proved to be very sympathetic, and the operation was performed under local spinal anesthesia, without any subsequent recurrence of the delusion. At the 2-month follow-up clinic appointment, she was still having flashbacks of the memories, which were precipitated particularly by medical programs on television and subsequent medical complications she had developed.

ICU support group—lessons learned

My awareness of the struggles patients and their families were having during the patients' recovery from critical illness grew with my work in the outpatient clinic and the results of the follow-up study. In 1994, we at Whiston Hospital decided to set up a patient and family support group. Initially, patients were invited to attend the support group several months after their discharge from ICU and only if they were known to be suffering psychological distress. But these patients proved hard to help in the group setting, as they were already exhibiting a fairly well-established pattern of poor coping behavior (e.g., alcohol abuse used as a self-treatment for depression). The move to an open invitation to all patients, as soon as they were discharged to the wards, to attend the support group largely seemed to circumvent this problem. Also, a move to using a private side room in the local pub rather than a room in the hospital increased patient and family attendance.[7] Many patients were initially reluctant to return to the hospital, but the pub was not threatening.

Many patients attending the support group seemed to need to understand why they had memories of hallucinations or paranoid delusions from their period of critical illness, to allow them to move on.[7] It became clear that such memories were having a major impact on psychological recovery.

ICU MEMORY TOOL

As part of my PhD research I designed an interview tool, the ICU Memory Tool, to assess patients' recall prior to ICU admission, during their critical illness, and after transfer to the general wards. The development phase involved the analysis of data collected in Whiston Hospital's post-ICU outpatient clinic, and this was combined with information gathered from in-depth semi-structured interviews with patients and their relatives. In the ICU follow-up clinic the simple questions "What do you remember of ICU?" and "Did you have any unpleasant memories" were asked of all patients, and their verbatim responses were recorded. The patients' statements were categorized at the time of collection using the following criteria applied by one researcher consistently over the years:

- Did the patient have any recall of his or her time in the ICU?
- If the patient had recall of actual events in the ICU, these were categorized and listed, for example, the presence of a nasogastric tube.

- Did the patient recall any nightmares (verified by description)?
- Did the patient recall any hallucinations (verified by description)?

Data from 159 patients attending our clinic at 2 months post-ICU were available for analysis, and the frequencies of particular memories were calculated. Of those 159 patients, 52% of patients reported not being able to remember anything about their stay in the ICU, 18% had no other memories but nightmares, and 4% could only remember hallucinations. We designed a semi-structured interview schedule using information from the analysis of the ICU outpatient data. Six patients and their closest relatives were approached to take part in in-depth semi-structured interviews of around 1 hour in duration. Three interviews took place with a relative present (with the permission of the patient) in order to examine the interaction between the patient and his or her relative. The other three interviews were with just the patient alone. Interviews were analyzed by identifying individual problems using content analysis for memories of the ICU. The information was pooled and used to construct the ICU Memory Tool.

I interviewed 45 patients about their memories of ICU 2 weeks after ICU discharge and assessed them for anxiety and depression using the Hospital Anxiety and Depression Scale (HADS). Three memory groups were found: those patients with no factual recall of the ICU but with what I called "delusional memories"—that is, hallucinations, nightmares, or paranoid delusions; those with factual recall and delusional memories; and those with no delusional memories. When anxiety scores were examined, it was the first memory group, those with no factual recall but with delusional memories, who scored most highly for anxiety (see Figure 1.1).[10] Acute posttraumatic stress disorder (PTSD)-related symptoms were assessed using the Impact of Event Scale (IES), and those patients who had no factual memories of the ICU but had delusional memories were also more likely to score highly for acute PTSD-related symptoms.[11]

INTERNATIONAL USE OF THE ICU MEMORY TOOL

The results from the ICU Memory Tool suggested that the presence of "delusional memories" was a powerful precipitant for anxiety and PTSD

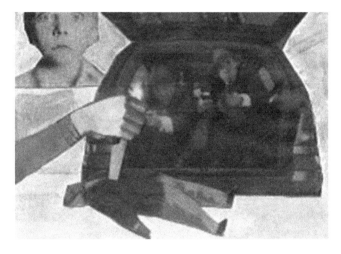

Figure 1.1. Collage illustrating patient's description of delusional memories of the ICU.

during the months following critical illness. The next step was to examine this in a larger multicenter study, and the RACHEL research group was born following a chance meeting at a European Society of Intensive Care Medicine (ESICM) Congress. A total of 238 patients across five ICUs in five European countries had their memories assessed using the ICU Memory Tool, and PTSD was assessed 3 months after ICU discharge. The factors found to be related to the development of PTSD were recall of "delusional memories," prolonged sedation, and physical restraint with no sedation. Those patients with a premorbid history of psychological problems—for example, previous depression or panic attacks—were likely to receive more sedation and recall delusional memories.[12]

How to reduce the psychological impact of delusional memories

Another chance meeting at an ESICM Congress led Whiston Hospital to adopt ICU diaries, using the model of Carl Bäckman.[13] As part of the PTSD study a record was kept of those patients receiving ICU diaries, and these patients seemed to have lower levels of PTSD symptoms. The next logical step was to test the effect of ICU diaries on the incidence of PTSD in a randomized controlled trial. The RACHEL (Raising Awareness, after Critical illness, of adverse Health Events in the Long-term) study group had grown by word of mouth, and 12 ICUs across six European countries joined the study. A total of 352 patients were randomized to the study at 1 month, and the incidence of new cases of PTSD was dramatically reduced in the intervention group compared to the control patients (5% vs. 13%). We finally had something that helped patients cope with their memories.[14]

TRAINING AS A THERAPIST

During the years of research into the psychological impact of critical illness, I realized that finding a clinical psychologist willing to see patients while they were in the ICU or on the general wards was very difficult. The normal reaction of a patient's general practitioner was to prescribe antidepressants rather than offer therapy.[15] To fill the gap, I retrained as a psychotherapist and started to provide counseling for patients, in the ICU, on the general ward, in their own homes, and on an outpatient basis as needed.[16] After a postgraduate qualification, I needed other courses to deal with patients' traumatic memories, particularly memories of frightening nightmares, hallucinations, and delusions. Eye movement desensitization and reprocessing (EMDR) proved to be especially helpful in reducing the impact of these frightening memories. Hypnotherapy training was also useful to aid relaxation for patients in the ICU or to create a safe space for those patients whose turbulent childhoods had made it impossible for them to think of a safe place from their past to allow EMDR. For some patients their frightening memories from the ICU were linked to childhood trauma, and therapy had to deal with both the childhood memories and the ICU ones (Case History 2).

CASE HISTORY 2

One female patient, aged 38, was admitted to the ICU following a pedestrian road traffic accident. In the ICU she was very agitated on weaning from sedation and at times had to be sedated further because of the agitation. On the general ward after discharge she had panic attacks and could not sleep. With time she revealed that her recall of the ICU was that she was made to watch her daughter being sexually abused and then was sedated to stop her from intervening. She was having frequent flashbacks of this memory, and as soon as she fell asleep she was having nightmares replaying it. She agreed to therapy and with time revealed that she had been sexually abused as a child. To process the frightening memories from the ICU, she had to work through the original trauma of childhood sexual abuse.

BACK TO A SUPPORT GROUP—ICUSTEPS

One of my ICU patients (K) who came for therapy expressed a wish to meet other patients who had been through critical illness. By that point the ICUsteps support group in Milton Keynes was well established, and other U.K. ICUs were looking at the model for their patients. Over K's therapy sessions she kept coming back to establishing a support group for ICU patients and families and felt it was something she would like to be involved with, to give something back for all the care she had received and to use her experience to help others. I got in touch with the Milton Keynes ICUsteps organizers and arranged a visit to a drop-in session for both myself and K. Following the visit, we decided to found the Cheshire and Mersey ICUsteps support group, with six weekly drop-in sessions of 2 hour's length. I wrote to all ICU patients from the previous year to find out who would be interested in attending the support group. We booked a local village hall, which had good transport links, a room available, and a kitchen to make tea and coffee. We put an advertisement on the ICU coffee room notice board asking if any staff would be interested in helping with the group. For the first group two other ICU nurses, K, and I were the founder members, and eight patients with three family members turned up. The topics discussed ranged widely, but memories of hallucinations and nightmares featured prominently. Over the next few drop-in sessions a group of patients and relatives was formed, and new patients and families were then able to attend.

NURSE, PARENT, AND RESEARCHER—RAMONA HOPKINS

July 11, 1981 was a hot summer day with blue sky and sunshine; it is a day I will never forget. We were barbequing with our neighbors in our back yard, and I remember thinking it was almost time to get ready to work the 3 to 11 P.M. shift as a nurse. I heard someone yelling that a child was pinned under our electric garage door. My husband went through the garage to try to force up the automatic garage door, and I ran into the house and called 911. I then heard yelling that it was our 4-year-old son; he was not breathing, and there was no pulse. I raced into the front yard and began cardiopulmonary resuscitation (CPR). Once the paramedics arrived they continued the CPR.

My son was taken by ambulance to the closest hospital and stabilized. He was then flown by helicopter to Primary Children's Medical Center in Salt Lake City. We were told that he had suffered severe anoxia, and the doctors did not know if he would live. He was sedated, mechanically ventilated, and admitted to the ICU, where he remained for most of the next 6 weeks. Eventually, things began to improve slowly, and he was extubated and began to breathe on his own, but he remained semi-comatose but stable for days and slowly became more alert. The day arrived when it was time for my son to be discharged, and his physician recommended that he be admitted to a long-term care center where the full-time care he required could be provided. His prognosis was uncertain, and it was unclear if he would walk or talk again, let alone attend school. The doctor offered to provide us a list of appropriate facilities that his condition warranted.

I was young and unprepared for the extreme challenges this brought. Even though I was a nurse and thought I knew what to expect, I was wrong. I was completely overwhelmed. My son came home, and he could not walk, talk, or care for himself. We had to feed him, change his diapers, carry him, dress him, and bathe him; he was completely dependent. My husband and I proceeded to start our son on a daily course of physical and cognitive rehabilitation that continued for years. During this time, I researched the rehabilitation literature and the effects of anoxia on the brain, trying to find therapies that would benefit him. I was surprised to learn that there was very little information regarding rehabilitation following anoxic brain injury. Further, the existing literature indicated that outcomes following anoxic brain injury were extremely poor. I was frustrated, but I was concerned about his recovery and trying to help him, so I returned to the university to study the effects of anoxic-ischemic injury on the brain and subsequently earned a PhD in psychology from the University of Utah.

My research was focused on the cognitive and psychological effects of anoxic-ischemic brain injury in individuals with cardiac and respiratory arrest or following carbon monoxide poisoning. My research also began to use brain imaging to assess the neuroanatomical effects of anoxic-ischemic brain injury via computed tomography (CT) and magnetic resonance imaging (MRI). Over time, my research broadened to include individuals who survived critical illness, including patients with acute respiratory distress syndrome (ARDS), patients with severe sepsis, and patients who were mechanically ventilated and experienced hypoxia-ischemia episodes during their critical illness.

Cognitive impairment following critical illness

In 1999 my colleagues and I published the first study that assessed cognitive outcomes in survivors of ARDS. We found that 100% of patients who survived ARDS had cognitive impairment at hospital discharge ($n = 55$). We followed these patients for a year, and at 1 year we found that 78% of patients had one or more impairments in memory, attention, concentration, and mental processing speed. In addition, the patients' overall intellectual functioning was lower than expected given their age and education level.[17] The cognitive impairments in these patients were associated with a longer duration of hypoxia while critically ill. In 2005, in a larger group of 74 ARDS survivors, we assessed cognitive impairment at hospital discharge and 1 and 2 years later.[18] Of these patients, 73% had cognitive impairments at hospital discharge, 46% had cognitive impairments at 1 year, and 47% had cognitive impairments at 2 years. The duration of hypoxemia during the critical illness was associated with impairments in verbal memory, attention, and executive function.[18] Thus, similar to what I found in studies in other disorders, survivors of ARDS experienced significant hypoxemia that was associated with cognitive impairments.

This study illustrates several factors replicated in subsequent studies: 1) a third to half of survivors of critical illness develop new cognitive impairments, and 2) in some patients, cognitive function improves over time, while other patients have persistent cognitive impairments that last years. One question this study did not address directly was whether cognitive impairments were new following critical illness or if they preceded the critical illness and were caused by other factors, such as pre-existing medical disorders. A number of subsequent studies have demonstrated that cognitive impairments after critical illness are indeed new, occurring or worsening after critical illness, such as the study by Iwashyna and colleagues in older adults surviving severe sepsis.[19] Further, cognitive impairments can persist years after hospital discharge, and they can occur in young, middle, and older age groups.[20] To date, no unique critical illness or intensive care pattern of deficits among cognitive impairments has been identified, as cognitive impairments occur in a wide variety of cognitive domains.[21] The cognitive impairments do not occur in a vacumn but, rather, unfavorably impact activities of daily living, functional outcomes (i.e., managing finances and medications, traveling and household chores), ability to return to work, and quality of life in survivors of critical illness.[18,22]

While the findings of cognitive impairments after critical illness have been replicated in small single-center cohort studies, three recent large multicenter studies confirmed that cognitive impairments post-ICU represent a substantial burden to patients and families. The ARDS Network Long-Term Outcomes Study (ALTOS), in which I was a co-principal investigator with Dr. Dale Needham at Johns Hopkins, assessed cognitive outcomes in the ARDSNetwork EDEN trial and found that 36% of survivors at 6 months and 25% of survivors at 12 months had cognitive impairments.[22] A second multicenter ALTOS study was an ancillary study to the Statins for Acutely Injured Lungs from Sepsis (SAILS) National Heart, Lung, and Blood Institute (NHLBI) clinical trial and assessed cognitive outcomes following the ARDSNetwork study comparing rosuvastatin to placebo for sepsis-associated ARDS.[23] There were 272 ARDS survivors, of whom cognitive impairment occurred in 37% at 6 months and 29% at 12 months.[23] In a separate large multicenter study from Vanderbilt University in which I was a co-investigator, in 871 survivors of critical illness, almost one third had cognitive impairments, and these were similar in severity to those found in patients with mild Alzheimer's disease or moderate traumatic brain injury.[20]

Post–intensive care syndrome

While the number of studies that assess critical illness and intensive care long-term outcomes is increasing rapidly, there is little consistency in the timing of outcome assessment, instruments used, and terminology and outcomes assessed. I was fortunate to be invited to be a member of the Society of Critical Care Medicine's Long-term Outcome Task Force. Over a period of several years, beginning in 2010, a group of stakeholders and ICU outcomes researchers met to discuss how to improve long-term outcomes for survivors of critical illness and their families.[24,25] The stakeholders reported that increased awareness and education regarding ICU outcomes was needed for patients, families, and care providers. We also identified barriers to optimal clinical practice as well as research gaps. An important result of the conference was the recognition that survivors experience a multitude of morbidities, usefully summarized with the term *post-intensive care syndrome* (PICS). *PICS* became the recommend term to describe new or worsening physical, cognitive, or psychological disorders after critical illness.[25] The use of a single term to describe the morbidities patients experience after critical illness has improved communication between patients and their families and care providers and has focused research on post-ICU outcomes. In addition, we recognized that family members of ICU patients could develop morbidities, including psychological morbidities such as depression and PTSD (these morbidities are summarized with the term *PICS-family*, or PICS-F).

A second stakeholder's conference was held in 2012, and the report of the conference was published in 2014. The focus of this conference was to improve patient and family outcomes by developing relevant strategies and resources.[24] At the second stakeholders' meeting we identified additional ways to improve outcomes after critical illness, including raising the awareness of, treatment for, and prevention of PICS; building institutional support for patients and families; and understanding and addressing barriers to optimal clinical practice.[24] The 2014 report emphasized that research was needed to better understand long-term physical, cognitive, and psychological outcomes, including studies designed to understand risk factors for PICS, mechanisms of injury, how to prevent PICS, optimal outcome measures and screening tools, and other potential interventions to improve patients' and families' quality of life.

Brain imaging following critical illness

I was also interested in understanding the effects of anoxic-ischemic injury on brain integrity. Previously in my research I had assessed neuroanatomical effects of traumatic brain injury, severe anoxia, and carbon monoxide poisoning using neuroimaging techniques. I was very interested in applying brain CT and MRI to assessment of ICU survivor populations. Early brain imaging studies used clinical scans and visual inspection or radiological reports to identify brain abnormalities (e.g., lesions, bleeding, atrophy, and other pathology) in ICU populations. Clinical brain imaging investigators have found that white matter lesions,[26] acute infarcts, and hemorrhage are common in critical illness populations.[27]

While this provided evidence that critical illness was associated with neuropathology, the studies were uncontrolled and retrospective. Thus I wanted to use quantitative neuroimaging techniques to assess structural injury in ICU populations. With my colleagues I conducted a retrospective study in 15 ARDS survivors in which we measured brain volumes and found significant ventricular enlargement and an increase in ventricle-to-brain ratio, suggesting brain atrophy in these patients.[28] Since the early studies, several other studies have found significant generalized atrophy, ventricular enlargement, sulcal widening, and, in some patients, hippocampal atrophy in survivors of critical illness.[29-32] One study found that patients who survived critical illness had greater hippocampal atrophy than did healthy controls.[33] White matter disruption (lower fractional anisotropy on diffusion tensor imaging) was also reported in the corpus callosum and internal capsule in ICU survivors.[34] The next step was to assess the relationship of atrophy to cognitive impairments. Investigators in several studies reported that cognitive impairments are associated with brain lesions, atrophy, and white matter damage.[33-37]

In sum, neuroimaging studies in ICU populations find diverse focal and global lesions and atrophy that are associated with cognitive impairments, which suggests that the brain injury is diffuse and a common problem after critical illness. While findings of neuronal injury or atrophy may be worrisome, neuroimaging provides opportunities to look for mechanisms of injury, design studies to prevent brain injury, assess the effectiveness of interventions, and develop compensatory strategies. Neuroimaging may allow for prognostication of outcomes and be used to guide post-ICU rehabilitation.

Improving cognitive outcomes

As we have learned more about PICS, research has begun to focus on preventing or improving PICS and PICS-F. As yet, few interventions have been tested in critical illness populations. While several studies have found that early mobility in the ICU decreases ICU and hospital lengths of stay,[38-41] there is little evidence so far that it improves long-term cognitive function in critically ill patients. However, results in other populations suggest that exercise or physical rehabilitation (including mobility) improves ability to complete activities of daily living, decreases depression and anxiety, and improves cognitive function.[42] Two small cohort studies assessed early mobility-based rehabilitation on cognitive impairments. Investigators in a study involving 87 critically ill patients randomized to usual care, once-daily physical therapy, or once-daily early physical therapy plus cognitive therapy found no difference in cognitive function across groups at 3 months.[43] Investigators in a within-subjects design cohort study in 637 neurological ICU patients found that an early exercise program in the ICU did not reduce depression or anxiety among ICU survivors.[38] However, in a prospective study of combined physical and cognitive rehabilitation post-ICU, clinical researchers found improved executive function in survivors of critical illness who had the intervention.[44]

I have also been privileged to be member of the Society of Critical Care Medicine's (SCCM's) THRIVE initiative, the goals of which are to support patients and families; educate patients, families, and clinicians; and focus on innovative research regarding recovery from critical illness, with an overall goal of improving outcomes after critical illness. As part of THRIVE, a Peer Support Collaborative has developed a network community to help meet the needs of survivors of critical illness through peer support. The Collaborative allows sharing of information across the network sites in order to develop peer support, share ideas, and develop best practices.[45] Models currently include support groups of ICU survivors, support of families while the patient is in the ICU, support in the hospital for patients and families, and the online support group. The SCCM and THRIVE initiative have awarded two grants so far to fund innovative research on the nature of recovery and survivorship. In addition, a website that contains information and videos on PICS and how to improve outcomes has been developed and is being expanded. Such novel strategies are desperately needed. Survivors are aware of the new cognitive deficits and other morbidities they are experiencing and are actively seeking information and interventions as they struggle to understand the changes in their lives. The THRIVE initiative provides a means to help survivors grapple with, come to understand, and accept the changes they experience after critical illness.

THE ICU PATIENT—PETER GIBB

Becoming an ICU patient

The last thing I remember from before my accident was going to see the group Placebo play at Brixton Academy, London, the night before, on April 23, 2003, and advising my friend to buy a concert T-shirt because he would never have the chance to do so again. That was my last memory before entering the ICU. I'm told I went to work the following day, put in a full day at the office, and left from there to go mountain biking with Mike, a colleague I worked and rode with regularly. We went to Aspley Woods, just outside Milton Keynes, UK, as usual for a training ride. We were both going to the French Alps in a couple of months' time for a week's riding holiday with some other friends, and we were in training to make sure we were in peak condition and ready to tackle the Free Raid Classic, a 40-mile Alpine bike ride we'd signed up for.

We reached the point on the ride where there was a fast downhill with a jump on it, which I'd done numerous times before, each time taking it a little faster and being airborne for a little further. I'm told that other riders had been digging around the jump, altering the angle of takeoff, but I took the jump anyway. Mike can't quite place what happened, and events rather took over. Something went wrong and soon after I'd left the ground, the bike and I parted company, and I landed head-first at full speed. Had I not been wearing my bike helmet as I always did, I'd almost certainly have been killed as I landed. The expanded polystyrene helmet did its job and shattered, taking the brunt of the impact. Even with this, I was left with a subarachnoid hemorrhage, a broken rib that gave me a bilateral pneumothorax with aspirated stomach contents, a fractured vertebra in my neck (C1), and two broken vertebrae in my back (compound fracture of T6 and T7). I was struggling to breathe and unable to move, but I've been told I was still conscious, though I lost consciousness before help arrived.

Mike couldn't get a signal on his mobile phone, so he rode quickly to the edge of the woods where he'd stand a better chance of summoning help. As luck would have it he happened across a resident of the village, Keith, who also happened to be a first-responder. They put the call in to emergency services and returned to where I was. Keith kept me still and warm and they waited for help. It was at this time that I lost consciousness. Dan, another mountain biker, happened on the scene and he, too, stayed to help. Given the remote location of the accident, the ambulance couldn't find me. Even if they had known where I was, there was no vehicular access, and it would have been a good 7- or 8-minute walk along the bridleway. Thankfully, the local air ambulance was called in, and, despite having been in the process of putting the helicopter away for the night at its home near Maidenhead, their paramedics were at my side in less than 15 minutes.

The paramedics gave me a chest drain on the spot and fitted me to the spinal board stretcher. Then all those present helped carry me down to the field where the helicopter had managed to land. They maneuvered me over the fence and loaded me into the air ambulance. Moments later they touched down at Milton Keynes General Hospital and I was taken to the emergency department.

Thanks to the diary my wife Mandy kept, I have a reasonable idea of how she found out, arriving home from her job late in the evening to find Mike and another colleague waiting outside the house. How she felt, however, I can't possibly imagine. From the accounts and stories I've heard from my family, I feel I have an idea as to the things that happened during my stay in intensive care, but I don't actually remember them. I remember the controls for raising and lowering the bed, and that I had to remember that one of the nurses was called Arnell, not Anselmo as I wanted to call him. I remember trying to scratch a letter to a band I was due to see in concert with a pen that didn't work; I was barely able to hold a pen, let alone write. The first real memory I had that things weren't right was the large pad of wadding over my throat where I'd had a tracheostomy. My sedation had been stopped several days before this, and I'd had conversations with staff and family members, but I only know these things from other people telling me about them. I have no recollection of them myself. To my perception, I went to bed one night, and when I woke up, nearly 3 weeks were missing and my life had been turned on its head.

Between the medication and the head injury my memory is patchy for events several months after this, although I remember some moments and feelings quite clearly. I don't remember the mood swings and depressions I'd sink into (which I've been told about subsequently), but I do remember the need to be able to see a clock from wherever I was. I wasn't convinced by the "stories" I'd been told, about my treatment, my injuries, and how I'd ended up where I was. It was like being trapped in a bizarre dream and very reminiscent of the plot of the film *The Matrix*.

My family members were told I had night terrors, though I only remember two dreams specifically. In one dream I was strapped to the underside of a German World War II fighter plane, along the length of its body, with my arms outstretched under the wings as it took off and flew. In the other dream I was on a restaurant boat in Hong Kong harbor, being chased and knocking over a wine glass. I'm also told I went through a Spanish-speaking phase, even though I don't speak Spanish. For the longest time I didn't know whether this was real or not, but I have since been reassured it was, despite my never having studied Spanish at that time.

I started physiotherapy and mobilization late in my ICU stay, and it was then that my physiotherapist noticed I was exhibiting clonus, and it became clear that my spinal injury was unstable. Suddenly, after starting to get better, I was put on bed rest and told to lie on my back at all times—I was not even allowed to cross my ankles!

I tried to make sense of everything around me, and the slightest inconsistency drew my attention, convincing me that this reality that I now found myself in was no more real than any other dream, although this seemed a quite vivid dream. Even something as small as a word could provide a clue as to this false reality around me. People were talking about a "tracheostomy," but I "knew" that to be wrong. In all the U.S. television programs, all I'd ever heard it called was "tracheotomy," no "s." Everyone seemed to accept this word without question, and I was the only one who spotted that it was wrong. This sense of unreality was only added to by the sudden change from getting better to having my physiotherapy stopped and my being held captive in bed.

Leaving the ICU

The move to the general ward was traumatic. Initially, the right sort of mattress couldn't be found for my spinal injury, though the staff found one eventually. The step-down of care from critical care to the general ward was more of a plummet. I felt like I'd just been dumped onto a general orthopedic ward. The staff had me down as being there for "rest and recuperation." No one seemed to know what I'd been through, what I was still going through, or what I would go on to face in my ongoing recovery. To begin with I had to be log-rolled, but following one particular shift change I could be assist-rolled, which was a positive sign of improvement. When the next shift change took place, however, it was back to being log-rolled. My treatment seemed worryingly haphazard.

I acted toward the medical staff like I was okay—bright, full of smiles, alert—trying to convince them to send me home, but when they weren't there I was withdrawn, preferred my curtains closed, and didn't want visitors outside the immediate family. I also developed an obsession with being able to see a clock, with the passage of time and with timekeeping more generally. If Mandy was later for her evening visit than I calculated she should be, I'd become very upset and agitated.

Paranoia

I avoided television programs and music I wasn't familiar with. I was scared that the plot lines and quality in this fake reality I thought I was in wouldn't be able to match the creativity I expected, and it would cause this dream world I was in to come crashing down around me.

I had no real perception of how seriously injured I'd been or how serious my ongoing condition was. I still fully expected to be going on my mountain biking vacation in a few months' time. It was only 2 weeks after my accident that the staff found that I had unstable compression fractures of two of my vertebrae and that there would, most likely, be spinal cord damage. Up to this time I'd even been gotten out of bed and had begun physiotherapy. When my consultant one day dismissively told me that I would have permanent spinal damage but only a foot drop, like the U.K. actor John Thaw, I was devastated. The idea that any serious damage, let alone permanent, had been done was like a thunderbolt. From being mobilized and getting better, I was now confined to my bed and not allowed to sit up, have my legs bent, or even cross my ankles. I was supposed to lie flat on my back, completely still for 3 weeks.

As time went on I became increasingly convinced that there was a conspiracy to keep me in that place. The rollercoaster of the way my injuries were discovered to be worse and how they were treated seemed to take me on a downturn after having improved, and this added weight to my belief in the conspiracy. One of the things I "knew" was that broken bones take 6 weeks to heal, and the spine would be no different. When 6 weeks were up, I would be out, or so I thought.

I understood that physiotherapy would be a necessary precursor to release, but I wouldn't be able to begin rehabilitation until I had my spinal brace. I remember when I was measured for it that the technician said it would be ready in "a few days." In my mind, that meant 3 days, no longer. When 3 days elapsed and there was still no spinal brace, it reinforced my belief that they were trying to keep me there. This belief deepened as reason after reason emerged as to why I needed to stay there longer. When my wife came in one Monday morning to try and find out from the doctor what was next in my treatment and was fobbed off with no answer, I was not surprised. I expected it, as their reasons for keeping me there were becoming more and more flimsy. I told my wife I wanted out and that I was leaving the hospital. I blackmailed her emotionally, telling her that if she did not help me, I would try to escape when she wasn't around and that I'd probably end up dead in a ditch somewhere. It took all my powers of persuasion to force her to help me, but eventually I convinced her. I regret having made her do that, inflicting the guilt that would follow, but to this day I'm grateful that she did help me, and I always will be.

Some sort of cloth corset with metal rods in it had appeared at the foot of my bed a day or two previously. I took this to be the spinal brace I was waiting for but that they had "forgotten" to tell me was there. In hindsight, I don't know what it was or how it got there, but it wasn't the spinal brace. Getting up for the first time in over 3 weeks, we strapped on the corset and, grasping the Zimmer frame that had been constantly by my bed-side the previous 3 weeks, I summoned reserves of strength I didn't know I had and began my escape. One condition Mandy had made me agree to was that I would tell them I was leaving. Naturally I agreed, as this was an obstacle to my escaping. As we reached the nurse at the desk by the exit I told her, as I'd agreed to do, that I was discharging myself. I recall her seeming flustered, which made sense to me, as I was not behaving as their plan would have me. She asked me to wait and speak to a doctor, and I calmly agreed but with absolutely no intention of doing so. I would not let them thwart my escape, not so close to getting out of their clutches. As soon as she went to get the doctor, I was off.

I'm not proud of what I did, especially not of what I forced my wife to do, and I regret that the management of my injuries and state of mind made this, to my mind, a "necessary" course of action. The idea of a man escaping the hospital in his pajamas with a Zimmer frame may seem almost as comical as it is bewildering and pathetic, but in the state of mind I was in, with what I'd been through, it was the only conceivable course of action. I've since had it explained to me by a brain injury specialist that it was actually quite under-standable, under my circumstances, that I took the only steps I could see to take control of my life again, however ill-advised those steps may have been.

After hospital discharge

In the early days at home, I was scared to go on my computer, for rea-sons similar to those for avoiding the music and television programs in the hospital. It was 3 weeks before I turned my computer on, and I was scared I wouldn't be able to do my job again, as I worked as a Web developer. I was also suffering from mood swings. After I'd been home for a few weeks, we would occasionally venture into town for a coffee. On one occasion, when we got back to the car, another car had parked too close to the passenger side for me to get in. I was so enraged, I spat on its windscreen. My moods were unpredictable and swung to extremes. I was frustrated at the length of time it took to recover. Throughout this period, both in the hospital and at home, time passed as slowly as it did when I was a child.

Brief suicide attempt

My anxiety, mood swings, and sense of disbelief came to a head one summer evening when I threw my Zimmer frame down on the patio in a fit of frustration. I still didn't believe this "reality" around me, and I'd had enough. I lurched down the drive with the intent of finding a car to step in front of and bring this fake life to an end. As I reached the road, a doubt niggled me. What if I was wrong? It would be so unfair to my wife and parents. So I decided to stay in this game for now and see how it played out, but I still didn't believe it was real. My suicidal episode lasted all of 5 minutes, but it was serious, and I had intent.

Revisiting the ICU

Revisiting the ICU helped start to convince me that perhaps this life I was now living was real. In talking to the follow-up nurse, I didn't feel like anything was being hidden from me. After one of the follow-up visits, I wanted to see the physiotherapy gym, of which I had a vague recollection. The journey to get there unwittingly took me past the orthopedic ward—which can best be described as my own personal Auschwitz. It's not a place I would have chosen to go, and I was shocked when I found myself there, but confronting this place took away the fear, power, and horror it represented in my mind.

Back to work

My first visit back to work was on the 7th of July. Even at this time, I was scared of seeing so many faces I was supposed to know and of being overwhelmed. So I stayed in the reception area while some of my colleagues came down to see me. This was followed 3 days later by a letter from the Personnel Department, saying I had to be back at work by mid-August or my salary would be stopped, despite 14 years' service.

My first official day back at work was August 7 (14 weeks after the accident); I was lucky with the timing. I wouldn't have chosen to return to work quite so soon, and it was mentally and physically challenging (I was still wearing the spinal brace and using the Zimmer frame), but it did force me to take another step back toward a normal life.

Orthopedic follow-up at the hospital

A couple of weeks after my escape, I had an appointment back at my hospital consultant's fracture clinic. It was the first time I'd left the house since arriving home. I remember how sweet the air smelled as I shuffled from the front door to the car. My paranoia was such that I went with my wife, my brother, and my sister-in-law because I genuinely feared the hospital staff would try to recapture me.

Community head injury clinic and my spinal injury

While on the general ward, my family had insisted I be seen by a brain injury nurse, because ward staff didn't seem to appreciate my condition, owing to my acting well. She also came and visited me at home and helped me to start to understand some of my thoughts. Far from condemning my escape, she understood it. She said it made sense because I was taking control of my life again.

I was referred to the community head injury clinic by the brain injury nurse. On my visits there I talked with and was assessed by the clinical psychologist, who helped reassure me I was normal. On later visits I saw the consultant in neurorehabilitation, and she was happy my head injury had recovered but noticed my walking wasn't right. She tested me for clonus, which was again present, so she referred me to Stoke Mandeville, the U.K. National Spinal Injuries Centre. After CT and MRI scans at Stoke Mandeville I was diagnosed with a kyphosis of T6 and T7, which required 10 hours in surgery to correct, with the fitting of a spinal fixator and a 3-week stay while I recovered.

My second life

A year to the day after my accident, I threw a party, inviting friends, family, colleagues, and medical staff (who'd helped save my life) to come and celebrate with me. It was, in a way, the first birthday of my second life.

Like the Warren Beatty film *Heaven Can Wait*, at quite an early stage in my recovery, I came to think of what had happened as the previous occupant of this body dying in the accident, and I was born into it. It almost came as a surprise when I had memories that must have belonged to the previous occupant.

Each memory was like a thread between these two lives, and the more memories I had, the more they knitted to form a gauze. The photographs I had from this time that I couldn't remember were like plaster over that gauze, helping to make a cast for these two disparate lives to join together.

The party was wonderful. Mo Peskett, my follow-up nurse, and her husband came, as did the pilot and one of the paramedics from the air ambulance that rescued me initially. It was good to be able to say thank you, and it was a real milestone in my recovery.

The ICU support group—ICUsteps

Later that year I received a letter from Mo inviting ex-ICU patients to a meeting to see if there was something we could do to help others going through similar experiences. I went along to see if I could help. Like many

ICU survivors, I felt a great desire to repay the debt of gratitude I owed to those who had saved me, and to give purpose to everything I had been through, by using those experiences to help others.

After a few meetings, we settled on the idea of holding drop-in sessions, where recent patients could come and talk to others who were further down the road of recovery, to help them realize they are not alone in what they feel and think and that, more often than not, what they're experiencing is normal for someone who has been through critical illness. Thus, ICUsteps was born.

We didn't know if others would feel the same as us, but we felt we had to try. It turned out we were right; visitors found it a great help to be able to talk about what they'd been through to people who understood them, having been through similar experiences themselves. As we say in ICUsteps, we provide empathy, not sympathy.

During my stay at Stoke Mandeville, I noticed a camaraderie among the spinal patient community, but I believe it's a theme with other illness groups too. Being treated in a specialist unit with people who have similar issues helped us support each other through adversity. Facing treatment and recovery together with others who are in the same boat really seemed to help, but I could see the contrast with ICU patients. As soon as we're no longer classified as "critically" ill, we can be bounced to anywhere in the hospital. Our chances of having the support of other survivors who can relate to what we've been through, or what lies ahead for us, is negligible, and this isolation from those like us makes coping harder.

It was hardly surprising in retrospect that the drop-in sessions worked. When we saw first-hand the difference they made to patient recovery, we just had to keep the group going. Mo and I co-authored an article,[46] which helped spark wider interest, and our first U.K. satellite group started in 2010. In 2016 the number of local groups was more than 20 and they continue to grow.

When we were contacted through our Website by a pair of nurses who were writing a patient information leaflet and asking for our thoughts, we were struck by the amount of effort likely being duplicated up and down the United Kingdom and decided to take this idea further. After extensive consultation with patients, relatives, and healthcare professionals, our booklet, "Intensive Care—A Guide for Patients and Relatives," was published in 2008. Despite negativity from some quarters, telling us that it wasn't needed and hospitals wouldn't adopt it, I'm pleased to say this was prediction unfounded. Healthcare professionals and companies seemed to recognize the value of patient information, in plain language and written by those who've been there. When my wife and I started work on that first draft back in 2006 while we were on vacation, we never dreamed it would end up growing into something widely seen as the U.K. standard for critical care patient information. Ten years on, we've printed around 150,000 copies, translated it into over 16 languages, and had it adapted for use in a dozen different countries around the world. We never dreamed at the outset that it would grow like this, but it's something all of us who've worked on the booklet are immensely proud of.

Speaking about the ICU

Back in 2005, Mo asked me if I would be willing to participate in a debate at an ICU follow-up conference on the pros and cons of taking photographs of ICU patients. She had seen the photographs my Dad had taken of me while I was in the ICU, and I was only too happy to help. She put me at ease by telling me that delegates at medical conferences always love the talks given by patients, and, after publication of the article we co-authored on support groups, we did some more presentations together. I had served as a patient representative on two U.K. National Institute of Clinical Excellence (NICE) clinical guideline committees, and, after CG83[47] had been launched, there were other invitations to speak on the patient experience of critical illness. As Mo once said, "The more you do, the more you do."

She was right; one thing led to the next, and over the years, I have spoken at over 50 conferences, meetings, and training days across the

United Kingdom and Europe—and this for someone who had never done any public speaking before and certainly doesn't regard himself as a natural speaker.

REFERENCES

1. Celsus AC. De Medicina. Approximately 47 CE.
2. Eisendrath SJ. ICU syndromes: their detection, prevention and treatment. *Crit Care Update*. 1980;7(4):5–8.
3. Dorr-Zegers O. Space and time in the intensive care unit. (Study of psychiatric problems which are seen in the ICU). *Actas Luso Esp Neurol Psiquiatr Cienc Afines*. 1988;16(4):246–254.
4. Jones C, Griffiths RD, Macmillan RR, et al. Psychological problems occurring after intensive care. *Br J Intensive Care*. 1994;2:46–53.
5. Griffiths RD, Jones C, Macmillan RR. Where is the harm in not knowing? Care after intensive care. *Clin Intensive Care*. 1996;7(3):144–145.
6. Compton P. Critical illness and intensive care: what it means to the client. *Crit Care Nurse*. 1991;11(1):50–56.
7. Jones C, Macmillan RR, Griffiths RD. Providing psychological support to patients after critical illness. *Clin Intensive Care*. 1994;5(4):176–179.
8. Jones C, Griffiths RD, Humphris G. A case of Capgras delusion following critical illness. *Intensive Care Med*. 1999;25(10):1183–1184.
9. Capgras J, Reboul-Lachaux J. L'illusion des ` sosies' dans un délire systématise chronique. *Bull Soc Clin Med Mentale*. 1923;2:6–16.
10. Jones C, Humphris GH, Griffiths RD. Preliminary validation of the ICUM tool: a tool for assessing memory of the intensive care experience. *Clin Intensive Care*. 2000;11(5):251–255.
11. Jones C, Griffiths RD, Humphris G, et al. Memory, delusions, and the development of acute posttraumatic stress disorder-related symptoms after intensive care. *Crit Care Med*. 2001;29(3):573–580.
12. Jones C, Bäckman C, Capuzzo M, et al. Precipitants of post-traumatic stress disorder following intensive care: a hypothesis generating study of diversity in care. *Intensive Care Med*. 2007;33(6):978–985.
13. Bäckman C, Jones C. Implementing a diary programme in your ICU. *ICU Manage*. 2011;11(3):10–16.
14. Jones C, Bäckman C, Capuzzo M, et al. Intensive care diaries reduce new onset post-traumatic stress disorder following critical illness: a randomised, controlled trial. *Crit Care*. 2010;14(5):R168.
15. Jones C, Griffiths RD. Patient and caregiver counselling after the intensive care unit: what are the needs and how should they be met? *Curr Opin Crit Care*. 2007;13(5):503-507.
16. Jones C, Hall S, Jackson S. Benchmarking a nurse-led ICU counselling initiative. *Nurs Times*. 2008;104(38):32–34.

17. Hopkins RO, Weaver LK, Pope D, et al. Neuropsychological sequelae and impaired health status in survivors of severe acute respiratory distress syndrome. *Am J Respir Crit Care Med*. 1999;160(1):50–56.
18. Hopkins RO, Weaver LK, Collingridge D, et al. Two-year cognitive, emotional, and quality-of-life outcomes in acute respiratory distress syndrome. *Am J Respir Crit Care Med*. 2005;171(4):340–347.
19. Iwashyna TJ, Ely EW, Smith DM, et al. Long-term cognitive impairment and functional disability among survivors of severe sepsis. *JAMA*. 2010;304(16):1787–1794.
20. Pandharipande PP, Girard TD, Jackson JC, et al. Long-term cognitive impairment after critical illness. *N Engl J Med*. 2013;369(14):1306–1316.
21. Wolters AE, Slooter AJ, van der Kooi AW, et al. Cognitive impairment after intensive care unit admission: a systematic review. *Intensive Care Med*. 2013;39(3):376–386.
22. Needham DM, Dinglas VD, Bienvenu OJ, et al. One year outcomes in patients with acute lung injury randomised to initial trophic or full enteral feeding: prospective follow-up of EDEN randomised trial. *BMJ*. 2013;346:f1532.
23. Needham DM, Colantuoni E, Dinglas VD, et al. Rosuvastatin versus placebo for delirium in intensive care and subsequent cognitive impairment in patients with sepsis-associated acute respiratory distress syndrome: an ancillary study to a randomised controlled trial. *Lancet Respir Med*. 2016;4(3):203–212.
24. Elliott D, Davidson JE, Harvey MA, et al. Exploring the scope of post-intensive care syndrome therapy and care: engagement of non-critical care providers and survivors in a second stakeholders meeting. *Crit Care Med*. 2014;42(12):2518–2526.
25. Needham DM, Davidson J, Cohen H, et al. Improving long-term outcomes after discharge from intensive care unit: report from a stakeholders' conference. *Crit Care Med*. 2012;40(2):502–509.
26. Suchyta MR, Jephson A, Hopkins RO. Brain MR and CT findings associated with critical illness. *Proceedings of the American Thoracic Society*. 2005;Abstracts 2:A426.
27. Sutter R, Chalela JA, Leigh R, et al. Significance of parenchymal brain damage in patients with critical illness. *Neurocrit Care*. 2015;23(2):243–252.
28. Hopkins RO, Gale SD, Pope D, et al. Ventricular enlargement in patients with acute respiratory distress syndrome. *J Int Neuropsychol Soc*. 2000;6:229.
29. Hopkins RO, Gale SD, Weaver LK. Brain atrophy and cognitive impairment in survivors of acute respiratory distress syndrome. *Brain Inj*. 2006;20(3):263–271.
30. Jackson JC, Hopkins RO, Miller RR, et al. Acute respiratory distress syndrome, sepsis, and cognitive decline: a review and case study. *South Med J*. 2009;102(11):1150–1157.
31. Gunther ML, Morandi A, Krauskopf E, et al. The association between brain volumes, delirium duration, and cognitive outcomes in intensive care unit survivors: the VISIONS cohort magnetic resonance imaging study. *Crit Care Med*. 2012;40(7):2022–2032.
32. Morandi A, Gunther ML, Vasilevskis EE, et al. Neuroimaging in delirious intensive care unit patients: a preliminary case series report. *Psychiatry (Edgmont)*. 2010;7(9):28–33.
33. Semmler A, Widmann CN, Okulla T, et al. Persistent cognitive impairment, hippocampal atrophy and EEG changes in sepsis survivors. *J Neurol Neurosurg Psychiatry*. 2013;84(1):62–69.

34. Morandi A, Rogers BP, Gunther ML, et al. The relationship between delirium duration, white matter integrity, and cognitive impairment in intensive care unit survivors as determined by diffusion tensor imaging: the VISIONS prospective cohort magnetic resonance imaging study*. *Crit Care Med.* 2012;40(7):2182–2189.

35. Brown CHt, Sharrett AR, Coresh J, et al. Association of hospitalization with long-term cognitive and brain MRI changes in the ARIC cohort. *Neurology.* 2015;84(14):1443–1453.

36. Hopkins RO, Gale SD, Weaver LK. Brain atrophy and cognitive impairment in survivors of acute respiratory distress syndrome. *Brain Inj.* 2006;20(3):263–271.

37. Jackson JC, Morandi A, Girard TD, et al. Functional brain imaging in survivors of critical illness: a prospective feasibility study and exploration of the association between delirium and brain activation patterns. *J Crit Care.* 2015;30(3):653.e1–653.e7.

38. Klein K, Mulkey M, Bena JF, et al. Clinical and psychological effects of early mobilization in patients treated in a neurologic ICU: a comparative study. *Crit Care Med.* 2015;43(4):865–873.

39. Morris PE. Moving our critically ill patients: mobility barriers and benefits. *Crit Care Clinics.* 2007;23(1):1–20.

40. Needham DM, Korupolu R. Rehabilitation quality improvement in an intensive care unit setting: implementation of a quality improvement model. *Top Stroke Rehabil.* 2010;17(4):271–281.

41. Titsworth WL, Hester J, Correia T, et al. The effect of increased mobility on morbidity in the neurointensive care unit. *J Neurosurg.* 2012;116(6):1379–1388.

42. Hopkins RO, Suchyta MR, Farrer TJ, et al. Improving post-intensive care unit neuropsychiatric outcomes: understanding cognitive effects of physical activity. *Am J Respir Crit Care Med.* 2012;186(12):1220–1228.

43. Brummel NE, Jackson JC, Girard TD, et al. A combined early cognitive and physical rehabilitation program for people who are critically ill: the activity and cognitive therapy in the intensive care unit (ACT-ICU) trial. *Phys Ther.* 2012;92(12):1580–1592.

44. Jackson JC, Clune H, Hoenig M, et al. The Returning To Everyday Tasks Utilizing Rehabilitation Networks (RETURN) Trial: a pilot feasibility trial including in-home cognitive rehabilitation of ICU survivors. *Am J Respir Crit Care Med.* 2010;181:A5359.

45. Mikkelsen ME, Jackson JC, Hopkins RO, et al. Peer support as a novel strategy to mitigate post-intensive care syndrome. *AACN Adv Crit Care.* 2016;27(2):221–229.

46. Peskett M, Gibb P. Developing and setting up a patient and relatives intensive care support group. *Nurs Crit Care.* 2009;14(1):4–10.

47. National Institute for Health and Care Excellence (NICE). Rehabilitation after critical illness in adults. Clinical guideline [CG83]. March 2009. Retrieved from https://www.nice.org.uk/guidance/cg83

Delirium in Critically Ill Patients

MARK VAN DEN BOOGAARD AND PAUL ROOD

DEFINITION OF DELIRIUM

Delirium is a psycho-organic disorder, implying that a physical cause underlies the cognitive dysfunction with psychological features. The *Diagnostic and Statistical Manual of Mental Disorders,* 5th ed. (DSM-5)[1] lists five main features that characterize delirium:

1. A disturbance in attention (reduced ability to direct, focus, sustain, and shift attention) and awareness
2. A disturbance in cognition (memory, orientation, language, visuospatial ability, or perception)
3. The disturbance develops over a short period of time (usually hours to days), represents a change from baseline, and tends to fluctuate during the course of the day.
4. The disturbance is not better explained by another pre-existing, evolving, or established neurocognitive disorder, and does not occur only in the context of a severely reduced level of arousal, such as coma.
5. There is evidence from the history, physical examination, or laboratory findings that the disturbance is caused by a medical condition, substance intoxication or withdrawal, or a medication side effect.

Additional features that may accompany delirium include the following:

6. Psychomotor behavioral disturbances such as hypoactivity, hyperactivity with increased sympathetic activity, and impairment in sleep duration and architecture
7. Variable emotional disturbances, including fear, depression, euphoria, or perplexity

OCCURRENCE

Delirium occurs frequently in hospitalized patients, but most frequently in critically ill patients in intensive care units (ICUs). In ICU patients, large differences in prevalences have been described, ranging between 11 and 89%.[2-4] This wide range can be explained by differences in ICU patient case-mix and methods of screening.[5] The median prevalence rate is around 30%.[6]

Delirium can be distinguished in three subtypes[7]:

1. Hyperactive subtype: the delirious patient is hyperalert or agitated
2. Hypoactive subtype: the delirious patient is hypoalert or lethargic
3. Alternating or mixed subtype: characterized by alternating hyperactive and hypoactive symptoms

The hyperactive subtype is characterized by motor agitation, including picking and pulling at catheters and tubes, and it is associated with delusions, hallucinations, and disorientation. It occurs in approximately 10% of patients with delirium, depending on the type of admission.[4] The hypoactive subtype, characterized by lethargy, psychomotor slowing and inappropriate speech or mood, occurs in approximately 35% of patients with delirium.[4] In intensive care patients with delirium, the alternating or mixed subtype is the most common, occurring in 60–70% of patients of delirium. The hypoactive subtype is more difficult to recognize without a formal assessment, and its incidence and prevalence are therefore likely underreported.

IMPACT OF ICU DELIRIUM

Delirium is associated with worse short- and long-term outcomes. Patients with delirium require longer periods of mechanical ventilation, have prolonged ICU and hospital stays with more frequent ICU readmissions, and more frequently remove tubes and catheters prematurely. These complications are independent of age and severity of illness.[4,8] It is unknown whether these short-term consequences are similar across patient categories and delirium subtypes.

In addition, patients with delirium have a significantly higher mortality rate than that of patients without delirium.[4,8–10] Importantly, for every day a patient is delirious, the mortality risk increases approximately 10%.[3,11] As noted in Chapter 3, the duration of delirium in the ICU is also important for patients' long-term cognitive functioning: the longer the duration, the worse their cognition.[12,13]

ASSESSMENT

The gold standard assessment for delirium includes an examination by a psychiatrist, neurologist, or geriatrician, who assesses delirium on the basis of DSM-5 criteria. In clinical ICU practice this is not feasible, especially considering delirium's fluctuating course, with worsening after sundown.[1,14] Thus, it is important for ICU clinicians to screen their patients using a delirium assessment tool. ICU nurses are optimal for delirium screening since, of all ICU clinicians, nurses spend the most time at patients' bedside and can closely observe their patients' behavior for long periods. Without a delirium assessment tool, nurses and physicians often fail to identify delirium, especially the hypoactive and the alternating subtypes.[15–17] Fortunately, several practical delirium assessment tools are now available for assessing ICU patients. Several ICU guidelines recommend that clinicians assess all ICU patients for delirium using a validated screening tool, preferably the Confusion Assessment Method for the ICU (CAM-ICU)[3,18] or the Intensive Care Delirium Screening Checklist (ICDSC).[19–23]

The CAM-ICU (Table 2.1) was originally developed and validated for use by ICU nurses in 2001.[3,18] The patient is examined for level of consciousness and cognitive functioning using a two-step approach. After determining the level of consciousness with, for example, the Richmond Agitation-Sedation Scale[24] or the Sedation-Agitation Scale,[25] the first feature to address is if there is an acute onset of mental status change or a fluctuating course. If a patient scores negative on this feature, delirium is absent. If this first feature is positive, the feature "attention, memory and

TABLE 2.1   CONFUSION ASSESSMENT METHOD FOR THE INTENSIVE CARE UNIT

Step 1 (mental status change): Is there an acute change in mental status from baseline, or has the mental status fluctuated over the last day?	If no: stop test—no delirium If yes: proceed to step 2
Step 2 (attention test): Ask the patient to squeeze your hand only when you say the letter *A*, then say the letters *SAVEAHAART* Alternative: picture test	If 2 errors or less: stop test— no delirium If 3 errors or more: proceed to step 3
Step 3 (level of consciousness): Assess level of sedation/agitation (using a validated tool like the RASS or SAS)	If RASS other than 0: stop test—delirium present If RASS 0: proceed to step 4
Step 4: Assess disorganized thinking: Ask: 1) Will a stone float on water? 2) Are there fish in the sea? 3) Does one pound weigh more than two? 4) Can you use a hammer to pound a nail? Then hold up two fingers, and ask the patient to imitate. As you lower your hands, ask the patient to repeat the action using the other hand, but do not demonstrate.	If 0–1 error: stop test—no delirium If more than 1 error: stop test—delirium present

RASS, Richmond Agitation-Sedation Scale;[24] SAS, Sedation-Agitation Scale;[25] Ely EW, Inouye SK, Bernard GR et al. (2001).[3]

focus" is tested. This can be done with an auditory test or a visual test, the latter developed by Hart et al.[26] If feature 2 is positive, level of consciousness (alert/calm, vigilant/hyperalert, lethargic, or stuporous) is assessed with feature 3. Feature 4 involves assessment of disorganized thinking. Only if features 1 and 2 plus 3 and/or 4 are positive is the patient assessed as delirious, according to the CAM-ICU.

The CAM-ICU can be administered in 2–3 minutes; however, members of the ICU team must be educated first in its use. Although originally the tool had a very high sensitivity of 95–100% and specificity of 93–98%[3] when performed by research nurses, its sensitivity appears lower (47%) in routine practice.[27] Overall, the pooled sensitivity is 80% (missing 20% of delirious patients), and the pooled specificity is 96% (meaning 4% of CAM-ICU positive results will be false positives).[28]

A drawback of the CAM-ICU is that it is a momentary test executed only once to three times a day. Given the fluctuating course of delirium, this can lead to false negative results. If the nurse or physician suspects delirium, the patient should be tested more frequently. Although there is no evidence regarding the optimal number of times a day patients should be screened, it is unlikely that assessing patients only once a day is sufficient. Also, the CAM-ICU cannot be used to quantify the severity of delirium[29] and does not address subsyndromal delirium.

The second recommended ICU delirium assessment tool, the ICDSC (Table 2.2), was developed by Bergeron et al.[19] The ICDSC is an observational instrument consisting of an eight-item checklist based on DSM-IV criteria. The eight items scored are altered level of consciousness, inattention, disorientation, hallucination/delusion/psychosis, psychomotor agitation or retardation, inappropriate speech or mood, sleep–wake cycle disturbance, and symptom fluctuation. These items are evaluated on the basis of observations made by the attending ICU nurse. If an item is present or positive, one point is scored. If a particular item cannot be assessed, it is rated as absent. A score of four or greater indicates a positive screen for delirium.

The first step of the ICDSC is assessment of the level of consciousness, using five categories (A–E). As with the CAM-ICU, in cases of no response

TABLE 2.2   INTENSIVE CARE DELIRIUM SCREENING CHECKLIST

Patient Evaluation	Points
Altered level of consciousness	
A: No response, *score none*	
B: Response to intense and repeated stimulation, *score none*	
C: Response to mild or moderate stimulation, *score 1*	
D: Normal wakefulness, *score 0*	
E: Exaggerated response to normal stimulation, *score 1*	
Inattention *(if yes, score 1; otherwise score 0)*	
Disorientation *(if yes, score 1; otherwise score 0)*	
Hallucination-delusion-psychosis *(if yes, score 1; otherwise score 0)*	
Psychomotor agitation or retardation *(if yes, score 1; otherwise score 0)*	
Inappropriate speech or mood *(if yes, score 1; otherwise score 0)*	
Sleep/wake cycle disturbance *(if yes, score 1; otherwise score 0)*	
Symptom fluctuation *(if yes, score 1; otherwise score 0)*	

Total score (0–8)
Score ≥4 = delirium
Score <4 = no delirium

From Bergeron N, Dubois MJ, Dumont M, Dial S, Skrobik Y. Intensive Care
Delirium Screening Checklist: evaluation of a new screening tool. *Intensive Care Med.*
2001;27(5):859–864.[19]

or the need for vigorous stimulation (category A or B), the patient is considered to be in a coma or stupor, and evaluation stops at that point. Category C scores one point for drowsiness or if mild to moderate stimulation is required for a response. Category D is wakefulness or a sleeping state from which the patient can easily be aroused, which is considered normal and scores no points. Hypervigilance is rated in category E, scoring one point.

The sensitivity of the test was found to be very high: 99% (with DSM-IV criteria as the reference standard), but the specificity was only 64%.[19] This implies that 36% of the patients identified as delirious with the ICDSC had false positive results. Based on a meta-analysis, the pooled sensitivity is 74% (26% false negatives), and the pooled specificity is 82% (18% false positives).[28]

Because this tool has an observational character, it doesn't have the disadvantage of limited screening moments during the day. A disadvantage of this observational tool is that patient's attention and performance are not necessarily tested as with the CAM-ICU. These important signs of delirium can be missed. Relevantly, the ICDSC assesses both the presence and the severity of delirium-related phenomena.

Future assessment of delirium

Authors of a systematic review with meta-analysis[28] recommended the use of either of these two screening tools. Notably, although both instruments have good screening properties, the delirium characteristics assessed differ greatly. Both methods of assessment have advantages and disadvantages. Testing some of a patient's cognitive functions is essential, as is longitudinal observation of a patient's behavior. Thus there is great potential in combining these and perhaps other tools to improve the performance of a delirium assessment.

Electroencephalography (EEG) can be very helpful for the diagnosis of delirium,[29-32] since delirium is a consequence of gross brain dysfunction. However, it is often not feasible to use 21-lead EEG monitors in critically ill patients. Also, a downside of EEG is the need for specialized personnel to measure and interpret the results. However, recent research suggests that a simplified EEG with automatic processing is technically feasible for the detection of delirium, and this technique may be suitable for daily practice.[29]

ETIOLOGY AND RISK FACTORS

The etiology of delirium is far from clear. A wide variety of factors are related to delirium, and the pathogenesis of delirium is typically multifactorial.[33-35]

Several neurotransmitter pathways have been implicated in delirium, including cholinergic, GABAergic, and serotonergic pathways.[34,36,37] Cytokines and glucocorticoids also appear relevant.[34,36,37] The cholinergic pathway, with acetylcholine as its neurotransmitter, plays a role in consciousness, and activation of cholinergic neurons is associated with dreaming, hallucinations,[38] and delirium.[37] The serotonergic pathway, with serotonin as the principal neurotransmitter, modulates mood, wakefulness, and cognition.[39] Benzodiazepines, alcohol, and some antibiotics activate GABA receptors, which can contribute to delirium. The inflammatory pathway also plays a role in delirium. For example, administration of the cytokine interleukin-2 can produce delirium.[40,41] In addition, it has become clear that other proinflammatory cytokines are associated with the onset of delirium in elderly[36] or critically ill[42] patients. The inflammatory pathway may be particularly important in critically ill patients, who often have systemic inflammation with sepsis, among other complications.

Critically ill patients often have many risk factors for delirium.[43] These risk factors can be divided into predisposing and precipitating factors. Predisposing factors include older age, heavy alcohol use, and history of cognitive disturbance. Precipitating factors include infection, hypoglycemia, pain, hypoxia, and the administration of restraints. In ICU patients, older age, dementia, hypertension, illness severity, recent delirium or coma, emergency surgery, mechanical ventilation, polytrauma, and metabolic acidosis are potent risk factors for delirium, while the use of dexmedetomidine instead of GABAergic medications is associated with reduced delirium.[44]

PREDICTION AND PREVENTION OF DELIRIUM IN INTENSIVE CARE PATIENTS

In view of the impact of delirium, there is a clear need for prevention, as well as for effective treatment. Prevention is likely most efficient and effective in ICU patients with the highest risk for developing delirium. To determine which patients have a high risk for delirium, a prediction model was recently constructed and validated, called the PRE-DELIRIC model.[45,46] The model contains 10 risk factors (age, Acute Physiology and Chronic Health Evaluation [APACHE-II] score, coma, admission category, infection, metabolic acidosis, morphine and sedative administration, urea concentration, and admission urgency) and can be used to predict the onset of delirium after 24 hours. Currently, an advanced model, The E-PRE-DELIRIC,[47] is being validated, in order to predict the chance for delirium at ICU admission.

Current guidelines emphasize nonpharmacological interventions to prevent delirium. These include early mobilization and environmental management, such as adapting light to the time of day and promoting nighttime sleep as much as possible.

Minimizing the use of sedative drugs is also important for delirium prevention. ICU practices are changing to ensure light or no sedation whenever feasible, so that patients are able to participate in early physical and occupational therapy.[48] Early rehabilitation reduces the incidence and duration of delirium, as well as muscle weakness, dependence on others, and time on the ventilator and in the ICU.[48]

Results of a before-and-after ICU delirium prophylaxis study suggest that administering low-dose haloperidol to those at high risk for delirium significantly reduces the incidence, prevalence, and complications of delirium.[49] A randomized controlled trial is currently under way to assess the safety and efficacy of haloperidol and other antipsychotics in this setting.

TREATMENT

The first step in treating delirium is to identify and eliminate potential contributing factors, including sepsis, shock, hypo- or hyperglycemia, electrolyte disorders, and hypoxia. It is also important to treat pain adequately, address drug withdrawal (including patients' psychiatric medications), and minimize deliriogenic medications as much as possible. Finally, it is important to promote adequate nighttime sleep, orient and mobilize the patient frequently, and minimize the use of physical restraints.

If delirium persists once identifiable causes have been eliminated, delirium treatment should include both nonpharmacological and pharmacological treatment strategies, with an emphasis on use of nonpharmacological interventions first.

Treatment strategies

Proven nonpharmacological treatments include the following:

1. Frequent reorientation, providing eyeglasses and hearing aids if needed
2. Maintaining sleep–wake cycles by minimizing environmental and procedural disturbances at night
3. Advancing mobility during the day as tolerated, with the ultimate goal of getting patients out of bed each day, even when they are mechanically ventilated

Pharmacological treatments include the following:

1. Adequate analgesia
2. Discontinuation of benzodiazepines (except when suspected ethanol or benzodiazepine withdrawal)
3. Resumption of psychiatric medications if indicated
4. Antipsychotics, if needed

The current guideline[21] has a limited number of recommendations on the use of antipsychotics for the management of delirium in ICU patients, primarily due to a lack of clear evidence for their safety and efficacy in this patient population. A recent review of the literature concluded that the pharmacological efficacy of antipsychotics for the treatment of ICU delirium is limited by "the small size of many studies, the inconsistency by which non-pharmacologic delirium prevention strategies were incorporated, the lack of a true placebo arm, and a failure to incorporate ICU and non-ICU clinical outcomes."[50] Nevertheless, antipsychotics, and haloperidol in particular, are commonly administered for the treatment of delirium in critically ill patients.[4]

In the future, sufficiently powered and carefully designed, multicenter, placebo-controlled trials are needed to determine the safety and efficacy of antipsychotics for the treatment of delirium in critically ill patients. Current guideline recommendations for the use of antipsychotics in the treatment of delirium are limited to the following:

1. Haloperidol for the treatment of delirium—*no recommendation,* due to a lack of evidence
2. Atypical antipsychotics *may* reduce the duration of delirium in ICU patients[51]
3. A strong recommendation *against* the use of rivastigmine (a cholinesterase inhibitor) for the treatment of delirium in ICU patients (based on a multicenter trial demonstrating that rivastigmine increased the severity and duration of delirium and the likelihood of death in these patients)[52]
4. A weak recommendation against the use of antipsychotics in patients with prolonged Q-T interval or other risk factors for torsades de pointes[21]

CONCLUSIONS

Delirium is very common in critically ill patients in the ICU, especially the mixed subtype (alternating hyperactivity and hypoactivity). The CAM-ICU and the ICDSC are useful delirium assessment tools in this setting. Several neurotransmitter pathways have been implicated in delirium, including cholinergic, GABAergic, and serotonergic pathways; cytokines and glucocorticoids also appear relevant. Risk factors for delirium in the ICU include older age, prior cognitive impairment, worse illness severity, recent delirium or coma, mechanical ventilation, admission category (especially trauma or neurological/neurosurgical admission), infection, metabolic acidosis, morphine and sedative administration, urea concentration, and admission urgency. Prevention and treatment of delirium should involve nonpharmacological interventions (frequent reorientation, providing eyeglasses and hearing aids if needed, promoting nighttime sleep, and early mobilization) and judicious use of opiate, sedative, and antipsychotic medications.

REFERENCES

1. American Psychiatric Association. *Diagnostic and Statistical Manual of Mental Disorders*. 5th ed. (DSM-5). Washington, DC: American Psychiatric Publishing; 2013.
2. Aldemir M, Ozen S, Kara IH, Sir A, Bac B. Predisposing factors for delirium in the surgical intensive care unit. *Crit Care*. 2001;5(5):265–270.
3. Ely EW, Inouye SK, Bernard GR, et al. Delirium in mechanically ventilated patients: validity and reliability of the confusion assessment method for the intensive care unit (CAM-ICU). *JAMA*. 2001;286(21):2703–2710.
4. van den Boogaard M, Schoonhoven L, van der Hoeven JG, van Achterberg T, Pickkers P. Incidence and short-term consequences of delirium in critically ill patients: a prospective observational cohort study. *Int J Nurs Stud*. 2012;49(7): 775–783.
5. van den Boogaard M, Pickkers P, Schoonhoven L. Assessment of delirium in ICU patients: a literature review. *Netherlands J Crit Care*. 2010;14(1):10–15.
6. Salluh JIF, Wang H, Schneider EB, et al. Outcome of delirium in critically ill patients: systematic review and meta-analysis. *BMJ*. 2015;350:h2538.
7. Peterson JF, Pun BT, Dittus RS, et al. Delirium and its motoric subtypes: a study of 614 critically ill patients. *J Am Geriatr Soc*. 2006;54(3):479–484.
8. Zhang Z, Pan L, Ni H. Impact of delirium on clinical outcome in critically ill patients: a meta-analysis. *Gen Hosp Psychiatry*. 2012;35(2):105–111.
9. Klein Klouwenberg PM, Zaal IJ, Spitoni C, et al. The attributable mortality of delirium in critically ill patients: prospective cohort study. *BMJ*. 2014;349:g6652.
10. Ely EW, Shintani A, Truman B, et al. Delirium as a predictor of mortality in mechanically ventilated patients in the intensive care unit. *JAMA*. 2004;291(14):1753–1762.
11. Pisani MA, Kong SY, Kasl SV, Murphy TE, Araujo KL, Van Ness PH. Days of delirium are associated with 1-year mortality in an older intensive care unit population. *Am J Respir Crit Care Med*. 2009;180(11):1092–1097.
12. Girard TD, Jackson JC, Pandharipande PP, et al. Delirium as a predictor of long-term cognitive impairment in survivors of critical illness. *Crit Care Med*. 2010;38(7):1513–1520.
13. van den Boogaard M, Schoonhoven L, Evers AW, van der Hoeven JG, van Achterberg T, Pickkers P. Delirium in critically ill patients: impact on

long-term health-related quality of life and cognitive functioning. *Crit Care Med.* 2012;40(1):112–118.

14. Duppils GS, Wikblad K. Patients' experiences of being delirious. *J Clin Nurs.* 2007;16(5):810–818.

15. Pandharipande P, Cotton BA, Shintani A, et al. Motoric subtypes of delirium in mechanically ventilated surgical and trauma intensive care unit patients. *Intensive Care Med.* 2007;33(10):1726–1731.

16. Inouye SK, van Dyck CH, Alessi CA, Balkin S, Siegal AP, Horwitz RI. Clarifying confusion: the confusion assessment method. A new method for detection of delirium. *Ann Intern Med.* 1990;113(12):941–948.

17. Spronk PE, Riekerk B, Hofhuis J, Rommes JH. Occurrence of delirium is severely underestimated in the ICU during daily care. *Intensive Care Med.* 2009;35(7):1276–1280.

18. Ely EW, Margolin R, Francis J, et al. Evaluation of delirium in critically ill patients: validation of the Confusion Assessment Method for the Intensive Care Unit (CAM-ICU). *Crit Care Med.* 2001;29(7):1370–1379.

19. Bergeron N, Dubois MJ, Dumont M, Dial S, Skrobik Y. Intensive Care Delirium Screening Checklist: evaluation of a new screening tool. *Intensive Care Med.* 2001;27(5):859–864.

20. Barr J, Fraser GL, Puntillo K, et al. Clinical practice guidelines for the management of pain, agitation, and delirium in adult patients in the intensive care unit. *Crit Care Med.* 2013;41(1):263–306.

21. Barr J, Pandharipande PP. The pain, agitation, and delirium care bundle: synergistic benefits of implementing the 2013 Pain, Agitation, and Delirium Guidelines in an integrated and interdisciplinary fashion. *Crit Care Med.* 2013;41(9 Suppl 1):S99–115.

22. van Eijk MMJ, Slooter AJC, Kesecioglu J, van der Mast RC. Delirium op de intensive care. *Ned Tijdschr Geneeskd.* 2008;152(51-52):2768–2773.

23. Dellinger RP, Levy MM, Carlet JM, et al. Surviving Sepsis Campaign: international guidelines for management of severe sepsis and septic shock: 2008. *Crit Care Med.* 2008;36(1):296–327.

24. Ely EW, Truman B, Shintani A, et al. Monitoring sedation status over time in ICU patients: reliability and validity of the Richmond Agitation-Sedation Scale (RASS). *JAMA.* 2003;289(22):2983–2991.

25. Riker RR, Picard JT, Fraser GL. Prospective evaluation of the Sedation-Agitation Scale for adult critically ill patients. *Crit Care Med.* 1999;27(7):1325–1329.

26. Hart RP, Levenson JL, Sessler CN, Best AM, Schwartz SM, Rutherford LE. Validation of a cognitive test for delirium in medical ICU patients. *Psychosomatics.* 1996;37(6):533–546.

27. van Eijk MM, van den Boogaard M, van Marum RJ, et al. Routine use of the confusion assessment method for the intensive care unit: a multicenter study. *Am J Respir Crit Care Med.* 2011;184(3):340–344.

28. Gusmao-Flores D, Salluh JI, Chalhub RA, Quarantini LC. The Confusion Assessment Method for the Intensive Care Unit (CAM-ICU) and Intensive Care Delirium Screening Checklist (ICDSC) for the diagnosis of delirium: a systematic review and meta-analysis of clinical studies. Crit Care. 2012; 16(4):R115.

29. van der Kooi AW, Zaal IJ, Klijn FA, et al. Delirium detection using EEG: what and how to measure. *Chest*. 2015;147(1):94–101.

30. Brenner RP. Utility of EEG in delirium: past views and current practice. *Int Psychogeriatr*. 1991;3(2):211–229.

31. Jacobson S, Jerrier H. EEG in delirium. *Semin Clin Neuropsychiatry*. 2000;5(2):86–92

32. Meagher DJ. Delirium: optimising management. *BMJ*. 2001;322(7279):144–149.

33. Fisch BJ, Spehlmann R. *Fisch and Spehlmann's EEG Primer: Basic Principles of Digital and Analog EEG*. 3rd ed. San Diego, CA: Elsevier; 1999.

34. Flacker JM, Lipsitz LA. Neural mechanisms of delirium: current hypotheses and evolving concepts. *J Gerontol A Biol Sci Med Sci*. 1999;54(6):B239–246.

35. Marcantonio ER, Rudolph JL, Culley D, Crosby G, Alsop D, Inouye SK. Serum biomarkers for delirium. *J Gerontol A Biol Sci Med Sci*. 2006;61(12):1281–1286.

36. de Rooij SE, van Munster BC, Korevaar JC, Levi M. Cytokines and acute phase response in delirium. *J Psychosom Res*. 2007;62(5):521–525.

37. Flacker JM, Cummings V, Mach JR, Jr., Bettin K, Kiely DK, Wei J. The association of serum anticholinergic activity with delirium in elderly medical patients. *Am J Geriatr Psychiatry*. 1998;6(1):31–41.

38. Perry EK, Perry RH. Acetylcholine and hallucinations: disease-related compared to drug-induced alterations in human consciousness. *Brain Cogn*. 1995;28(3):240–258.

39. DeNoble VJ, Schrack LM, Reigel AL, DeNoble KF. Visual recognition memory in squirrel monkeys: effects of serotonin antagonists on baseline and hypoxia-induced performance deficits. *Pharmacol Biochem Behav*. 1991;39(4):991–996.

40. Denicoff KD, Rubinow DR, Papa MZ, et al. The neuropsychiatric effects of treatment with interleukin-2 and lymphokine-activated killer cells. *Ann Intern Med*. 1987;107(3):293–300.

41. Rosenberg SA, Lotze MT, Yang JC, et al. Experience with the use of high-dose interleukin-2 in the treatment of 652 cancer patients. *Ann Surg*. 1989;210(4): 474–484.

42. van den Boogaard M, Kox M, Quinn KL, et al. Biomarkers associated with delirium in critically ill patients and their relation with long-term subjective cognitive dysfunction; indications for different pathways governing delirium in inflamed and noninflamed patients. *Crit Care*. 2011;15(6):R297.

43. Ely EW, Siegel MD, Inouye SK. Delirium in the intensive care unit: an under-recognized syndrome of organ dysfunction. *Semin Respir Crit Care Med*. 2001; 22(2):115–126.

44. Zaal IJ, Devlin JW, Peelen LM, Slooter AJ. A systematic review of risk factors for delirium in the ICU. *Crit Care Med*. 2015;43(1):40–47.

45. van den Boogaard M, Pickkers P, Slooter AJ, et al. Development and validation of PRE-DELIRIC (PREdiction of DELIRium in ICu patients) delirium prediction model for intensive care patients: observational multicentre study. *BMJ*. 2012;344:e420.

46. van den Boogaard M, Schoonhoven L, Maseda E, et al. Recalibration of the delirium prediction model for ICU patients (PRE-DELIRIC): a multinational observational study. *Intensive Care Med*. 2014;40(3):361–369.

47. Wassenaar A, van den Boogaard M, van Achterberg T, et al. Multinational development and validation of an early prediction model for delirium in ICU patients. *Intensive Care Med.* 2015;41(6):1048–1056.

48. Schweickert WD, Pohlman MC, Pohlman AS, et al. Early physical and occupational therapy in mechanically ventilated, critically ill patients: a randomised controlled trial. *Lancet.* 2009;373(9678):1874–1882.

49. van den Boogaard M, Schoonhoven L, van Achterberg T, van der Hoeven JG, Pickkers P. Haloperidol prophylaxis in critically ill patients with a high risk for delirium. *Crit Care.* 2013;17(1):R9.

50. Devlin JW, Al-Qadhee NS, Skrobik Y. Pharmacologic prevention and treatment of delirium in critically ill and non-critically ill hospitalised patients: a review of data from prospective, randomised studies. *Best Pract Res Clin Anaesthesiol.* 2012;26(3):289–309.

51. Devlin J, Skrobik Y, Riker R, et al. Impact of quetiapine on resolution of individual delirium symptoms in critically ill patients with delirium: a post-hoc analysis of a double-blind, randomized, placebo-controlled study. *Crit Care.* 2011;15(5):R215.

52. van Eijk MM, Roes KC, Honing ML, et al. Effect of rivastigmine as an adjunct to usual care with haloperidol on duration of delirium and mortality in critically ill patients: a multicentre, double-blind, placebo-controlled randomised trial. *Lancet.* 2010;376(9755):1829–1837.

Critical Illness and Long-Term Cognitive Impairment

RAMONA O. HOPKINS, MARIA E. CARLO,
AND JAMES C. JACKSON

INTRODUCTION

Cognitive impairment affects more than half of patients who survive critical illness in the United States.[1] Undiscriminating, cognitive impairment occurs in patients of all ages, previously healthy or not, and regardless of the type of critical illness or intensive care unit (ICU) in which they are treated. Cognitive impairment can be devastating to patients and their families. In a qualitative study by Cox and colleagues, in which patients and caregivers completed semi-structured interviews about their ICU experiences, a spouse noted, "It was like I was married to somebody else . . . he didn't remember anything I told him. I had to make lists for everything."[2] Cognitive impairment is associated with anxiety, depression, reduced health-related quality of life, inability to return to work, impairments in activities of daily living (e.g., bathing, toileting, dressing), and new deficits in ability to do instrumental activities of daily living (e.g., managing money, medications, and household chores).[3-8] Data suggest that some patients will regain some cognitive function within the first 12 months after ICU discharge, and the gains observed are often appreciable, although almost half of those with initial cognitive impairment have impairments that persist years after ICU discharge and are likely permanent.[9]

Critical illness and intensive care factors are underrecognized as risk factors for developing cognitive impairment. Understanding brain injury due to critical illness has the potential to elucidate pathways that lead to cognitive impairment, which in turn may drive effective preventive and therapeutic efforts. In this chapter, we review the prevalence, characteristics, possible mechanisms, and risk factors for long-term cognitive impairment (LTCI) after critical illness.

PREVALENCE OF COGNITIVE IMPAIRMENT

As we have noted elsewhere, cognitive impairment is strikingly widespread after critical illness, occurring in 11% to 62% of survivors, depending on the population evaluated and the cognitive tests administered (tests vary substantially in difficulty and quality).[1] A brief review of specific findings from studies conducted to date is illustrative. Among survivors of acute respiratory distress syndrome (ARDS), 70–100% had cognitive impairment at hospital discharge, 46–80% at 1 year, 20% to 47% at 2 years, and 20% at 5 years.[1] In a large prospective cohort study of 821 surgical and medical ICU patients that included adults of all ages, Pandharipande and colleagues found that 12 months after hospital discharge, one in four survivors had cognitive impairment similar in severity to that of patients with mild Alzheimer's disease, and one in three had impairment similar to that of patients with moderate traumatic brain injury.[8] Importantly, only 6% of the patients had cognitive impairment at baseline, which suggests that processes occurring during critical illness and intensive care interventions led to cognitive impairment. Data supporting the role of critical illness in cognitive impairment come from Iwashyna and colleagues, who examined cognitive function before and after severe sepsis in a large prospective cohort study of older persons. The authors found that individuals who survived severe sepsis had greater than three times higher odds of developing moderate to severe cognitive impairment compared to individuals who did not develop severe sepsis.[10] Thus the cumulative data from these studies show that cognitive impairment is a consistent finding across studies in ICU survivors, regardless of the etiology of their critical illness.

While the majority of studies have been small single-center studies, recently, larger multicenter studies have been conducted. In a multicenter ancillary study of the EDEN trial, conducted in 41 hospitals in the United States, 525 ARDS survivors were randomized to initial low-energy permissive feeding or to full-energy enteral feeding and completed cognitive screening tests at 6 and 12 months.[6] Cognitive impairment was present in 25% and 21% of survivors at 6- and 12-month follow-up, respectively, on the cognitive screening test; however, there was no difference in cognitive function between the two feeding groups.[6] In a related study involving 174 patients from 12 hospitals at five centers who completed a full battery of neuropsychological tests, investigators found that 36% and 25% of survivors had cognitive impairment at 6- and 12-month follow-up, respectively.[7] The cognitive impairments occurred in executive function, memory, verbal reasoning, attention, and working memory.[7] These findings were similar to those in a prior multicenter ARDS Network trial, in which survivors had impairments in verbal reasoning, memory, and word finding at 1-year follow-up.[11] A multicenter ancillary study of the ARDS Network trial that compared rosuvastatin versus placebo in ARDS patients with sepsis ($n = 272$) found that 37% of patients at 6 months and 29% at 12 months had significant cognitive impairments.[12] While there was no difference in cognitive impairments between the treatment groups, rosuvastatin was associated with worse delayed memory.[12] Finally, a large multicenter study from the Vanderbilt group on survivors of critical illness found that 40% had cognitive impairments at 3 months and 34% at 12 months.[8]

Cognitive impairment after critical illness involves multiple domains of cognition—most commonly attention, concentration, memory, and executive function, but also processing speed, visual-spatial abilities, and word-finding abilities. The most commonly reported impairments are in memory and executive function. For example, an analysis of the data from the BRAIN ICU study found that 26% of patients had impairments in executive function at 3 months on a questionnaire and 27% had impairments on the Trail Making Test Part B, a neuropsychological measure of executive function.[8] Impairments in executive function were independently associated with depression and worse quality of life at 12 months and age did not modify these associations.[8] Importantly, as in traumatic brain injury survivors, there is no "signature" cognitive profile observed in critical illness survivors, likely owing to the diffuse nature of the brain injury. There is nothing equivalent in critical illness survivor populations to the more specific patterns observed in Alzheimer's disease, for instance, where isolated deficits in memory occur in the disease's early states and are highly suggestive of the diagnosis. The impaired cognitive domains likely reflect combined factors—specific features of a critical illness and its treatment, along with individual vulnerabilities such as genetics, older age, and prior cognitive impairment. The trajectories of cognitive impairment over time are unclear due to a paucity of data—almost none pertaining to longitudinal functioning over extended time periods. There are likely multiple trajectories of cognitive functioning after critical illness and possibilities include (a) stable impairment, (b) improvement without complete recovery, (c) complete recovery, (d) improvement and then subsequent decline over time, and (e) stable normal cognition (no impairment). Currently, no predictive models can be applied to individual survivors of critical illness.

Differences in the prevalence of cognitive impairment across studies appear to be due in part to the use of cognitive screening tests instead of more comprehensive neuropsychological test batteries; comprehensive neuropsychological test batteries are more sensitive to detection of cognitive impairment, as implied.[6,7] In a study of 103 survivors of chronic critical illness, 29% and 25% had significant cognitive impairment as measured by the Mini Mental Status Examination (MMSE),[14] but the prevalence likely would have been higher if the investigators had administered a more comprehensive battery. Interestingly, the long-term prognostic value of in-hospital MMSE scores appears limited in critical illness survivors; Woon and colleagues found that MMSE scores at hospital discharge were not predictive of cognitive impairment at 6-month follow-up, as measured with a detailed neuropsychological test battery.[13] In the ARDS Network Long Term Outcomes Study (ALTOS), employing data from the Awakening and Breathing Controlled Trial (ABC), the MMSE had poor sensitivity (19–37%) cross-sectionally in detecting cognitive impairment assessed using neuropsychological tests.[14] While individuals with very low MMSE scores may genuinely be impaired (with the proviso that MMSE performance can generally be poor in normal elderly individuals with very limited education), a "normal" score on the MMSE does not rule out the presence of cognitive impairment. The somewhat inconsistent findings with the MMSE described have been reported elsewhere. For example, the MMSE has demonstrated good sensitivity and specificity in identifying mild cognitive impairment or dementia in older adults.[15] However, in cardiac and bariatric surgery patients, the ability of the MMSE to identify cognitive impairment is poor.[16,17] Data to date suggest that the MMSE is not a good tool to use in ICU populations, given its poor sensitivity in this population.

PATIENTS' PERCEPTIONS OF COGNITIVE IMPAIRMENTS

While most studies have used either cognitive screening tests or standardized neuropsychological test batteries, one study assessed the ICU survivor's perception of cognitive impairments using the Functional Assessment of Cancer Therapy—Cognitive Function (FACT-Cog) at 3 and 6 months after ICU discharge.[18] The FACT-Cog assesses four areas: (1) perceived cognitive impairments, (2) comments from others, (3) perceived cognitive abilities, and (4) interference with quality of life. Survivors of critical illness reported significantly higher levels of perceived cognitive impairments, reported that others were more likely to view them as impaired, and believed that their impairments interfered with their quality of life at 3 and 6 months.[18] Patients reported significant increases in cognitive impairments on the FACT-Cog after critical illness compared to their baseline ratings. Patients and family members were grouped into those who reported cognitive impairments and those without cognitive impairments. In the group with cognitive impairments, their baseline scores did not differ from the group without cognitive impairments; however, the cognitive impairment group had higher scores (new cognitive impairment) 3 months after ICU discharge. Pre-existing cognitive impairment at baseline was a risk factor for developing post-ICU cognitive impairment.[18]

"REAL-WORLD" EXAMPLES: CASE STUDIES OF COGNITIVE IMPAIRMENT AFTER THE ICU

Cognitive impairment has been widely observed in dozens of research studies, yet this impairment has typically been reflected in abnormal performance on neuropsychological testing batteries and rarely evaluated in the context of its "real-world" impact. However, if impairment is sufficiently severe to be considered clinically significant, then it will almost always result in actual functional consequences. Two recent brief examples, derived from our clinical work, demonstrate the ways that "real-world" impairment is expressed:

1. Driving: Mr. Smith was an 87-year-old veteran of World War II who experienced a long and complex critical illness which involved a 20-day ICU hospitalization. Prior to his critical illness, he was a high-functioning individual who, despite his advanced age, was fully independent. Upon his return home, he started driving again (about 3 weeks after discharge) and got into two consecutive accidents, even though he had never been in an auto accident before. While physically weak, his primary difficulty had to do with deficits in his ability to sustain attention and focus his attention on important things (i.e., road signs, stop lights, etc.) while at the same time ignoring nonessential and irrelevant distractions. His limitations became so severe and accelerated so rapidly that his family sold his car to prevent him from being on the road.

2. Employment: Mrs. Jones was a 36-year-old business person, a highly successful entrepreneur who was known for her impeccable judgment and her emotional intelligence. She developed ARDS and was hospitalized for approximately 3 weeks in the ICU, during which time she was delirious and on a mechanical ventilator. After discharge, she was eager to return to work, despite some evidence of deficits in her social functioning. She attended a crucial business meeting and, while there, appeared to have difficulty tracking the comments of others, while saying a number of inappropriate things that reflected a clear lack of inhibition (as well as a striking lack of self-awareness and critical reflection). Her employers were concerned that she was now a liability to their company and she was subsequently fired from her job.

While we have provided just two examples here, many more could be described, including those involving deficits in managing money and doing taxes and in learning how to use medical devices. Unfortunately, clinical providers are often unaware of these difficulties unless they ask about them specifically, as patients are often reluctant to talk about them. Querying patients about the nuanced ways that their cognitive impairment impacts their functioning is a very important practice and should increasingly become a routine feature of all clinical interactions with ICU survivors.

IS COGNITIVE IMPAIRMENT NEW OR PRE-EXISTING?

Critical illness is virtually always an unexpected event, so data on baseline cognitive functioning are not available in most studies (that is, patients cannot be tested beforehand, unlike patients undergoing elective surgery). Thus, it has sometimes been difficult to determine the extent to which cognitive impairment after critical illness is new or reflects a worsening of already existing impairment. Nevertheless, the mean age of most critically ill cohorts studied to date is approximately 54 years[1]; on average, these patients are 10 to 15 years younger than most patients with new-onset dementia. This suggests that a majority of the many thousands of people studied did not suffer from Alzheimer's disease or related conditions at the time of their ICU admissions. In addition, most cognitive outcome studies have screened participants for pre-existing neurocognitive impairment and have excluded patients with disorders associated with cognitive impairment (e.g., traumatic brain injury, stroke, dementia, and cardiovascular disease) based on patient or surrogate interview and chart review.[1] A few studies have used surrogate questionnaires to screen for pre-existing cognitive impairment.[6,7,19,20]

Some studies of older adults have used existing databases that assessed cognitive function serially, prior to, and after a critical illness and ICU admission, thereby providing baseline data to which cognitive function after critical illness could be compared (Table 3.1). One of these studies was mentioned previously, a nationally representative cohort study that used data from the Health and Retirement Study, which is a representative sample of elderly individuals in the United States in which cognitive and functional outcomes were assessed longitudinally. In this study, an episode of severe sepsis was independently associated with a more than three times higher odds of developing moderate to severe cognitive impairment[10]—that is, odds of developing cognitive impairment increased from 6.1% before to 16.7% after severe sepsis. The cognitive impairments remained at the next assessment 2 years later.[10] Similarly, Guerra and colleagues studied Medicare beneficiaries and found that 18% of patients who were treated in an ICU in 2005 had a new diagnosis of dementia within 3 years.[21] Risk factors associated with dementia included infection, acute neurological dysfunction, and acute need for dialysis.[21] In a follow-up study of Medicare beneficiaries treated in an ICU in 2005, Guerra and colleagues noted that a new diagnosis of dementia occurred in 15% of survivors over a 3-year period, compared to 12% in age-, sex-, and race-matched controls from the general population. The risk of receiving a diagnosis of dementia was 40% higher in the elderly patients who had survived critical illness, after accounting for known dementia risk factors.[22]

TABLE 3.1   STUDIES USING DATABASES TO ASSESS COGNITIVE IMPAIRMENT BEFORE AND AFTER CRITICAL ILLNESS HOSPITALIZATION

Study	Study Design	Sample Characteristics	Sample Size	Baseline Cognitive Impairments	Post-Critical Illness Cognitive Impairments
Iwashyna et al., 2010[10]	Prospective cohort study	Health and Retirement Study (1998–2008) Alive to at least one post-hospitalization follow-up survey	516 survivors of severe sepsis 4517 survivors of non-sepsis hospitalization to at least 1 follow-up survey	6.1% moderate to severe cognitive impairments before severe sepsis No change in cognitive impairment without severe sepsis	16.7% moderate to severe cognitive impairments after severe sepsis
Guerra et al., 2012[21]	Retrospective cohort study of Medicare standard Analytic Files data	5% random sample of Medicare beneficiaries who received intensive care in 2005 3-year follow-up	25,386 treated in the ICU and survived to hospital discharge	Excluded all patients with an ICD-9-Cm code for dementia, mild cognitive impairment, symptoms of general mental loss, cardiac surgery, or history of cardiac surgery	17.8% new diagnosis of dementia after critical illness Infection, severe sepsis, neurologic dysfunction, and acute dialysis were independently associated with diagnosis of dementia
Guerra et al., 2015[22]	Retrospective cohort study of Medicare standard Analytic Files data	2.5% sample of Medicare beneficiaries age 66 years or older in 2005 Matched population controls 3-year follow-up	10,348 ICU survivors	Excluded all patients with an ICD-9-Cm code for dementia, mild cognitive impairment, symptom of general mental loss and cardiac surgery or history of cardiac surgery	15% new diagnosis of dementia in ICU survivors and 12.2% in controls 3% increased absolute risk of a new diagnosis of dementia after accounting for risk factors for dementia

(continued)

TABLE 3.1 CONTINUED

Study	Study Design	Sample Characteristics	Sample Size	Baseline Cognitive Impairments	Post–Critical Illness Cognitive Impairments
Ehlenbach et al., 2010[50]	Prospective cohort study	Data from the Adult Changes in Thought study (1994–2007) Evaluated once every 2 years	1601 with no hospitalization 1287 with one or more noncritical illness hospitalization 41 with one or more critical illness hospitalization	93.2 (SD 4.7) 92.9 (SD 4.7) 93.9 (SD 4.4) (baseline Cognitive Abilities Screening Instrument scores)	mean 1.83 point decline mean 3.81 point decline mean 5.28 point decline Critical illness associated with greater cognitive decline
Iwashyna et al., 2012[51]	Retrospective cohort study of 1996–2008 Medicare Provider Analysis and Review files	Fee-for-service Medicare beneficiaries aged 65 and older with severe sepsis from 1998–2008 3-year follow-up	637,867 patients who survived severe sepsis for at least 3 years		Estimated moderate to severe cognitive impairment in 106,311 (95% CI 79,692–133,930) by 2008 (based on Iwashyna et al., 2010 data)

ICD-9, *International Classification of Disease*, Ninth Edition; ICU, intensive care unit; SD, standard deviation.

Nevertheless, it does not follow that critical illness causes a progressive form of cognitive impairment (like dementia with Alzheimer's disease). Rather, critical illness may cause a one-time decrement in cognitive functioning that can persist. It is also possible that post-ICU cognitive impairment can trigger dementia in an individual who did not have any prior symptoms of dementia, by accelerating the person's cognitive decline or loss of cognitive reserve.

As noted previously, Pandharipande and colleagues conducted a prospective cohort study of surgical and medical ICU patients of all ages, and they found that one in four patients had cognitive impairment similar in severity to that of patients with mild Alzheimer's disease, while one in three had impairments similar to moderate traumatic brain injury, 12 months after hospital discharge. Importantly, cognitive impairment occurred in both older and younger patients.[8] Thus, it would be incorrect to assume that only the elderly are at risk for critical illness–related cognitive impairment. While the severity of critical illness–related cognitive impairment is similar to that of patients with dementia, there are differences between the disorders. Similarly, critical illness–related delirium and long-term cognitive impairment are not identical. Table 3.2 compares cognitive impairments in patients with Alzheimer's disease, delirium, and long-term critical illness–related cognitive impairment.

MECHANISMS OF LONG-TERM COGNITIVE IMPAIRMENT

Multiple mechanisms appear to drive the development of cognitive impairment in survivors of critical illness, including dysregulation of metabolism such as hypoxia, hypotension, glucose dysregulation (hyperglycemia, hypoglycemia, and glucose variability), and hyperuremia. Hypoxia damages the brain through a number of biochemical mechanisms, including excitotoxic damage due to excitatory amino acid neurotransmitter release (e.g., glutamate), decreased adenosine triphosphate production, calcium influx, reperfusion and reoxygenation injury, apoptosis, necrosis,

TABLE 3.2 COMPARISON OF CHARACTERISTICS OF ALZHEIMER'S
DISEASE, DELIRIUM, AND LONG-TERM COGNITIVE IMPAIRMENT
AFTER CRITICAL ILLNESS

	Alzheimer's Disease	Delirium	Long-term Cognitive Impairment Post-ICU
Precipitants	Infection	Medication Acute medical problem Environmental change	Sepsis Acute respiratory failure ICU duration >24 hours with mechanical ventilation
Mechanisms of injury: Inflammation Hypoxia Ischemia Glucose Dysregulation	IL-1β, TNF-α Hypoxia Reduced cerebral blood flow Impaired glucose metabolism	IL-6, IL-8 associated with postoperative delirium Hypoxia Ischemia Reduced regional cerebral blood flow Hyperglycemia and hypoglycemia	Severe sepsis IL-6, IL-8, TNF-α Hypoxia Hypotension Hypoglycemia, hyperglycemia, and glucose variability
Risk factors	Older age Diabetes Obesity Depression Low physical activity Low mental activity Smoking Apolipoprotein e4 Hypertension Alcoholism Prior brain injury	Older age Sensory impairment Cognitive impairment Fewer years of education Apolipoprotein e4 Hypertension Alcoholism	Delirium Sedation

Clinical Characteristics

	Alzheimer's Disease	Delirium	Long-term Cognitive Impairment Post-ICU
Onset	Gradual onset over years	Acute onset, waxing and waning	Acute onset during hospitalization, often not recognized due to confounds of medications, delirium, weakness, and lack of cognitive evaluation

(continued)

TABLE 3.2   CONTINUED

	Alzheimer's Disease	Delirium	Long-term Cognitive Impairment Post-ICU
Cognitive domains affected	Memory the first to be affected, followed by impairments in executive function, processing speed, language, and motor skills	Attention and short-term memory	Memory Executive function Visuospatial reasoning Attention
Natural history	Gradual progressive decline; prognosis 10 years	Reversible by treating the underlying problem	Improvement during first 6 months to 1 year in some individuals Mild to severe deficits persist for years after critical illness
Associated functional impairment	Impairments in instrumental activities of daily living Unable to return to work Reduced quality of life	Impairments in instrumental activities of daily living during episode, which is normally time-limited and occurs during acute medical illness	Impairments in instrumental activities of daily living Unable to return to work Reduced quality of life

IL-1β, interleukin-1-beta; IL-6, interleukin-6; IL-8, interleukin-8; TNF-α, tumor necrosis factor alpha.

inflammation, and blood vessel endothelial damage.[23] While data are limited in critical illness survivor populations, Hopkins and colleagues found that a longer duration of hypoxemia was associated with cognitive impairment in ARDS survivors.[4] Supportive data come from a prospective multicenter study in which hypoxemia was independently associated with cognitive impairment 12 months after ARDS.[24] Hypoxia is associated with moderate to severe brain atrophy and enlargement of the temporal horns of the lateral ventricles in ARDS survivors, with concomitant memory impairment, suggesting damage to the medial temporal lobes.[25,26]

Cerebral vascular damage via hypotension and variations in cerebral blood flow is another mechanism of brain injury. Cortical and subcortical hypoperfusion in patients with critical illness is associated with cognitive deficits.[27] Hopkins and colleagues found that duration of hypotension with ARDS was associated with cognitive impairment at hospital discharge.[4] Similarly, Mikkelsen and colleagues found that lower central venous pressure was associated with cognitive impairment in ARDS survivors.[24] Postmortem studies in patients with septic shock show ischemic neuronal damage in a number of brain areas, including the hippocampus.[27]

The brain is also sensitive to disturbances in glucose supply,[28,29] and hypoglycemia causes neuronal death in widely distributed brain regions, including the hippocampus, cerebral cortex, and striatum.[30] Glucose dysregulation, including hypoglycemia, hyperglycemia, and blood glucose variability, during critical illness is associated with cognitive impairment.[30,31] Hopkins and colleagues found that moderate hyperglycemia and blood glucose variability predicted cognitive impairment 12 months after ARDS.[30] Similarly, in a surgical ICU population, one or more hypoglycemic events and blood glucose fluctuations were associated with cognitive impairment at 1-year follow-up.[31] Glucose accumulation in the brain contributes to apoptosis (programmed cell death).[29]

Inflammation is a well-described mechanism of brain injury in critically ill patients, especially patients with sepsis. Systemic inflammation can disrupt the blood–brain barrier and allow proinflammatory cytokines (intereukin-6 and C-reactive protein) to enter the brain.[32] One contributor to brain injury is upregulation of inflammatory mediators, including tumor necrosis factor alpha and interleukins (such as IL-6), which activate the complement cascade.[33] Data from rodents show that inflammation induces apoptosis in brain regions such as the hippocampus, a structure critical for memory.[34] Increased S100 calcium-binding protein B (S100B) and neuron-specific enolase, markers of neuronal injury, occur in patients with sepsis and are associated with cognitive impairment.[35] Furthermore, systemic inflammation is associated with whole-brain atrophy in survivors of critical illness.[36] These mechanisms (hypoxia, hypotension, glucose dysregulation, and inflammation) may further interact with risk factors such as older age and comorbid illness to enhance the risk of cognitive decline. Ultimately, the mechanisms described can lead to cellular dysfunction and may ultimately result in necrosis and apoptosis.

RISK FACTORS ASSOCIATED WITH COGNITIVE IMPAIRMENT

Current data suggest that critical illness–related cognitive impairment is not associated with age, smoking, alcohol misuse, or critical illness etiology or severity (e.g., Acute Physiology and Chronic Health Evaluation II score upon ICU admission, tidal volume, duration of mechanical ventilation, ICU length of stay, or days receiving sedative, narcotic, or paralytic medications).[37] Nevertheless, critical illness–related delirium is a well-described risk factor for long-term cognitive impairment, increasing the odds 12.5 times.[8,38] As described in Chapter 2, delirium is an acute disturbance of consciousness with inattention accompanied by a change in cognition or perceptual disturbance that fluctuates over time[39]; importantly, this syndrome occurs in up to 70% of critically ill patients.[40] Delirium has been associated with incident dementia independent of important confounders, such as age, sex, comorbid illness, severity of illness, or sedative or analgesic medication use.[38] In the large and definitive BRAIN-ICU study, a longer duration of delirium was associated with worse long-term global cognitive and executive function, independent of sedative or analgesic medication use, age, preexisting cognitive impairment, coexisting disease, and severity of illness in the ICU.[8] The duration of delirium is associated with impairments in memory and language 18 months after hospital discharge.[45] In mechanically ventilated critically ill patients duration of delirium was associated with new disability in instrumental activities of daily living.[47] Finally, a magnetoencephalography (MEG) study found desynchronization of brain function after sepsis compared to age-matched healthy controls that was associated with cognitive impairment, thought to be due to change in the interaction between brain regions.[47]

As the population ages, a growing number of people will develop cognitive impairment. Traditional risk factors studied include age, genetic factors (e.g., apolipoprotein E4), vascular risk factors (hypertension, hyperlipidemia, diabetes, and tobacco smoking), midlife obesity, and lifestyle factors (social, mental, and physical activity). The apolipoprotein E4 allele is associated with increased risk for cognitive impairment following traumatic brain injury,[41] carbon monoxide poisoning,[42] or cerebrovascular disease;[43] it is also associated with development of Alzheimer disease.[44] However, it remains unclear if the APOE4 allele is a risk factor for cognitive impairment following critical illness.

The impact of depression on cognition in survivors of critical illness remains largely unknown. As noted in Chapter 4, depression is common after critical illness, occurring in over a third of general medical and surgical ICU survivors in the first year after critical illness.[20] Interestingly, depression and cognitive impairment share some common risk factors in critical illness survivors, such as lower intelligence, hypoglycemia, and sedative use. In addition, cognitive impairment is a common manifestation of depression, especially in late-life depression. There may be cases of post-ICU cognitive impairment in which the cognitive impairment is a manifestation of depression. Alternatively, depression may be a consequence of cognitive and other sequelae of critical illness, including functional impairment, loss of employment, physical limitations, increased dependence on caregivers, and financial distress.

IMPLICATIONS OF COGNITIVE IMPAIRMENT

The impact of critical illness–related cognitive impairment on individuals and society is understudied. A qualitative study of 23 survivors of critical illness reported that the participants had new disability that interfered with activities of daily living, including new cognitive deficits that persisted months after leaving the hospital.[2] Both the patients and their caregivers stated that being critically ill affected all aspects of their lives. Cox and colleagues[2] reported that the "deleterious impact of cognitive deficits on patients' daily life we observed was underappreciated and sometimes dismissed by physicians." Cognitive impairment influences survivors' independence in instrumental activities of daily living (IADL; financial management, medication management, shopping, home care, etc.). In a prospective cohort study of 58 critically ill trauma survivors, 22% had IADL dependencies, and cognitive impairment was strongly associated with these dependencies.[45]

Health-related quality of life (HRQOL) is frequently reduced in survivors of critical illness compared to population norms[3,4,46] Unfortunately, the effect of critical illness–related cognitive impairment on HRQOL remains unclear; in two studies, no association was evident.[47,48] However, cognitive impairment has been shown to be associated with impaired HRQOL in populations of patients with other medical conditions, including stroke, trauma, traumatic brain injury, human immunodeficiency virus, carbon monoxide poisoning, chronic obstructive pulmonary disease, and liver transplantation.

Although the economic burden associated with critical illness–related cognitive impairment has not been estimated, it is likely substantial. For example, Rothenhausler and colleagues found that cognitive impairment in ARDS survivors was associated with inability to return to work.[49] In addition, patients with the level of cognitive impairment found in critical illness survivors often require many hours of caregiving per week.

FUTURE DIRECTIONS

While there is broad agreement that cognitive deficits can develop after critical illness, much remains to be learned. For example, relatively little is known regarding the trajectories of change in the months and years after ICU discharge. Clearly, a subset of patients—young as well as old— have persistent cognitive deficits, yet our clinical experience suggests that some patients get better and, indeed, transition to "normal" after initially displaying profound decrements. Significantly more needs to be learned about these "improvers," with the hope that insights about their experiences may one day inform clinical practice. Broadly speaking, future research efforts will likely benefit from a more intentional focus on the dynamics—whether genetic, clinical, or social—that contribute to thriving after critical illness instead of merely surviving. Other areas of future focus include the development of animal models to elucidate mechanisms of critical illness–related cognitive impairment and ways to harness neuroplasticity in cognitively impaired survivors.

SUMMARY

Cognitive impairment is a public health problem of great significance, found not only in persons with Alzheimer's disease and other dementing illnesses but in the millions of critical illness survivors around the world. Evidence from dozens of studies of thousands of individuals, many done with significant methodological rigor, suggests that up to one in two survivors of critical illness experience significant deficits in memory, executive functioning, attention, and processing speed. Some key risks factors—notably, delirium—may be modifiable, whereas others may not be modifiable. Efforts need to be directed not only at modifying risk factors but also at attempting to prevent, treat, and remediate deficits, as with other populations experiencing acquired brain injuries. These efforts will be aided by three developments:

1) *Increased research.* Clinical investigators at a handful of
   academic medical centers currently conduct most of
   the research in this area. We hope that this research will
   proliferate in future years and will take on a comprehensive
   and programmatic quality in which basic, translational,
   and clinical investigations will develop at centers dedicated
   primarily to post-ICU outcomes. Our hope is that this
   research will one day help to significantly alleviate the
   considerable suffering that unfolds daily in the lives of

brain-injured critical illness survivors and those who care most about them.

2) *Interdisciplinary involvement.* The magnitude of the public health problem of critical illness–related cognitive impairment is still largely underappreciated across healthcare disciplines, including clinical fields best equipped to address the cognitive issues discussed herein, namely psychology, neuropsychiatry, neurology, and rehabilitation medicine. But we need even broader expertise to thoughtfully tackle this issue, one of the great problems of our time.

3) *Integration of patient perspectives.* Consistent with our research culture's current emphasis, it will continue to be crucially important to integrate ICU survivors and their family members into the development of research and clinical interventions aimed at improving cognitive impairment. Few studies of post-ICU outcomes have integrated such individuals, and yet their insights into the nature of the impairment they experience and the ways that this impacts them adversely are vitally important.

REFERENCES

1. Wilcox ME, Brummel NE, Archer K, Ely EW, Jackson JC, Hopkins RO. Cognitive dysfunction in ICU patients: risk factors, predictors, and rehabilitation interventions. *Crit Care Med.* 2013;41(9 Suppl 1):S81–98.
2. Cox CE, Docherty SL, Brandon DH, et al. Surviving critical illness: acute respiratory distress syndrome as experienced by patients and their caregivers. *Crit Care Med.* 2009;37(10):2702–2708.
3. Herridge MS, Tansey CM, Matte A, et al. Functional disability 5 years after acute respiratory distress syndrome. *N Engl J Med.* 2011;364(14):1293–1304.
4. Hopkins RO, Weaver LK, Collingridge D, Parkinson RB, Chan KJ, Orme JF, Jr. Two-year cognitive, emotional, and quality-of-life outcomes in acute respiratory distress syndrome. *Am J Respir Crit Care Med.* 2005;171(4):340–347.
5. Jackson JC, Mitchell N, Hopkins RO. Cognitive functioning, mental health, and quality of life in ICU survivors: an overview. *Psychiatr Clin North Am.* 2015;38(1):91–104.

6. Needham DM, Dinglas VD, Bienvenu OJ, et al. One year outcomes in patients with acute lung injury randomised to initial trophic or full enteral feeding: prospective follow-up of EDEN randomised trial. *BMJ*. 2013;346:f1532.

7. Needham DM, Dinglas VD, Morris PE, et al. Physical and cognitive performance of patients with acute lung injury 1 year after initial trophic versus full enteral feeding. EDEN trial follow-up. *Am J Respir Crit Care Med*. 2013;188(5):567–576.

8. Pandharipande PP, Girard TD, Jackson JC, et al. Long-term cognitive impairment after critical illness. *N Engl J Med*. 2013;369(14):1306–1316.

9. Wolters AE, Slooter AJ, van der Kooi AW, van Dijk D. Cognitive impairment after intensive care unit admission: a systematic review. *Intensive Care Med*. 2013;39(3):376–386.

10. Iwashyna TJ, Ely EW, Smith DM, Langa KM. Long-term cognitive impairment and functional disability among survivors of severe sepsis. *JAMA*. 2010;304(16):1787–1794.

11. Mikkelsen ME, Shull WH, Biester RC, et al. Cognitive, mood and quality of life impairments in a select population of ARDS survivors. *Respirology*. 2009;14(1):76–82.

12. Needham DM, Colantuoni E, Dinglas VD, et al. Rosuvastatin versus placebo for delirium in intensive care and subsequent cognitive impairment in patients with sepsis-associated acute respiratory distress syndrome: an ancillary study to a randomised controlled trial. *Lancet Respir Med*. 2016 Mar;4(3):203–212. doi:10.1016/S2213-2600(16)00005-9. PubMed PMID: 26832963.

13. Woon FL, Dunn CB, Hopkins RO. Predicting cognitive sequelae in survivors of critical illness with cognitive screening tests. *Am J Respir Crit Care Med*. 2012;186(4):333–340.

14. Pfoh ER, Chan KS, Dinglas VD, et al. Cognitive screening among acute respiratory failure survivors: a cross-sectional evaluation of the Mini-Mental State Examination. *Crit Care*. 2015;19:220.

15. Lin JS, O'Connor E, Rossom RC, Perdue LA, Eckstrom E. Screening for cognitive impairment in older adults: A systematic review for the U.S. Preventive Services Task Force. *Ann Intern Med*. 2013;159(9):601–612.

16. Burker EJ, Blumenthal JA, Feldman M, et al. The Mini Mental State Exam as a predictor of neuropsychological functioning after cardiac surgery. *Int J Psychiatry Med*. 1995;25(3):263–276.

17. Galioto R, Garcia S, Spitznagel MB, et al. The Mini-Mental State Exam (MMSE) is not sensitive to cognitive impairment in bariatric surgery candidates. *Surg Obes Relat Dis*. 2014;10(3):553–557.

18. Baumbach P, Meissner W, Guenther A, Witte OW, Götz T. Perceived cognitive impairments after critical illness: a longitudinal study in survivors and family member controls. *Acta Anaesthesiol Scand*. 2016 Sep;60(8):1121–1130. doi:10.1111/aas.12755. Epub 2016 Jun 20. PMID: 27324080.

19. Jackson JC, Hart RP, Gordon SM, et al. Six-month neuropsychological outcome of medical intensive care unit patients. *Crit Care Med*. 2003;31(4):1226–1234.

20. Jackson JC, Pandharipande PP, Girard TD, et al. Depression, post-traumatic stress disorder, and functional disability in survivors of critical illness in the BRAIN-ICU study: a longitudinal cohort study. *Lancet Respir Med*. 2014;2(5):369–379.

21. Guerra C, Linde-Zwirble WT, Wunsch H. Risk factors for dementia after critical illness in elderly Medicare beneficiaries. *Crit Care.* 2012;16(6):R233.
22. Guerra C, Hua M, Wunsch H. Risk of a diagnosis of dementia for elderly Medicare beneficiaries after intensive care. *Anesthesiology.* 2015;123(5):1105–1112.
23. Johnston MV, Nakajima W, Hagberg H. Mechanisms of hypoxic neurodegeneration in the developing brain. *Neuroscientist.* 2002;8(3):212–220.
24. Mikkelsen ME, Christie JD, Lanken PN, et al. The adult respiratory distress syndrome cognitive outcomes study: long-term neuropsychological function in acute lung injury survivors. *Am J Respir Crit Care Med.* 2012;185(12):1307–1315.
25. Bigler ED, Blatter DD, Anderson CV, et al. Hippocampal volume in normal aging and traumatic brain injury. *AJNR Am J Neuroradiol.* 1997;18(1):11–23.
26. Yokota H, Ogawa S, Kurokawa A, Yamamoto Y. Regional cerebral blood flow in delirium patients. *Psychiatry Clin Neurosci.* 2003;57(3):337–339.
27. Sharshar T, Annane D, de la Grandmaison GL, Brouland JP, Hopkinson NS, Francoise G. The neuropathology of septic shock. *Brain Pathol.* 2004;14(1):21–33.
28. Pulsinelli WA, Jacewicz M, Levy DE, Petito CK, Plum F. Ischemic brain injury and the therapeutic window. *Ann N Y Acad Sci.* 1997;835:187–193.
29. Auer RN, Siesjo BK. Hypoglycaemia: brain neurochemistry and neuropathology. *Baillieres Clin Endocrinol Metab.* 1993;7(3):611–625.
30. Hopkins RO, Suchyta MR, Snow GL, Jephson A, Weaver LK, Orme JF. Blood glucose dysregulation and cognitive outcome in ARDS survivors. *Brain Inj.* 2010;24(12):1478–1484.
31. Duning T, van den Heuvel I, Dickmann A, et al. Hypoglycemia aggravates critical illness-induced neurocognitive dysfunction. *Diabetes Care.* 2010;33(3):639–644.
32. Nishioku T, Dohgu S, Takata F, et al. Detachment of brain pericytes from the basal lamina is involved in disruption of the blood-brain barrier caused by lipopolysaccharide-induced sepsis in mice. *Cell Mol Neurobiol.* 2009;29(3):309–316.
33. Bone RC. The pathogenesis of sepsis. *Ann Intern Med.* 1991;115(6):457–469.
34. Semmler A, Okulla T, Sastre M, Dumitrescu-Ozimek L, Heneka MT. Systemic inflammation induces apoptosis with variable vulnerability of different brain regions. *J Chem Neuroanat.* 2005;30(2-3):144–157.
35. Nguyen DN, Spapen H, Su F, et al. Elevated serum levels of S-100beta protein and neuron-specific enolase are associated with brain injury in patients with severe sepsis and septic shock. *Crit Care Med.* 2006;34(7):1967–1974.
36. Lindlau A, Widmann CN, Putensen C, Jessen F, Semmler A, Heneka MT. Predictors of hippocampal atrophy in critically ill patients. *Eur J Neurol.* 2015;22(2):410–415.
37. Hopkins RO, Jackson JC. Long-term neurocognitive function after critical illness. *Chest.* 2006;130(3):869–878.
38. Witlox J, Eurelings LS, de Jonghe JF, Kalisvaart KJ, Eikelenboom P, van Gool WA. Delirium in elderly patients and the risk of postdischarge mortality, institutionalization, and dementia: a meta-analysis. *JAMA.* 2010;304(4):443–451.
39. Meagher D, Trzepacz PT. Phenomenological distinctions needed in DSM-V: delirium, subsyndromal delirium, and dementias. *J Neuropsychiatry Clin Neurosci.* 2007;19(4):468–470.

40. McNicoll L, Pisani MA, Zhang Y, Ely EW, Siegel MD, Inouye SK. Delirium in the intensive care unit: occurrence and clinical course in older patients. *J Am Geriatr Soc.* 2003;51(5):591–598.

41. Li L, Bao Y, He S, et al. The association between apolipoprotein E and functional outcome after traumatic brain injury: a meta-analysis. *Medicine (Baltimore).* 2015;94(46):e2028.

42. Hopkins RO, Weaver LK, Valentine KJ, Mower C, Churchill S, Carlquist J. Apolipoprotein E genotype and response of carbon monoxide poisoning to hyperbaric oxygen treatment. *Am J Respir Crit Care Med.* 2007;176(10):1001–1006.

43. Perna L, Mons U, Rujescu D, Kliegel M, Brenner H. Apolipoprotein E e4 and cognitive function: a modifiable association—results from two independent cohort studies. *Dement Geriatr Cogn Disord.* 2015;41(1-2):35–45.

44. Bigler ED, Lowry CM, Kerr B, et al. Role of white matter lesions, cerebral atrophy, and APOE on cognition in older persons with and without dementia: The Cache County, Utah, study of memory and aging. *Neuropsychology.* 2003;17(3):339–352.

45. Jackson JC, Obremskey W, Bauer R, et al. Long-term cognitive, emotional, and functional outcomes in trauma intensive care unit survivors without intracranial hemorrhage. *J Trauma.* 2007;62(1):80–88.

46. Timmers TK, Verhofstad MH, Moons KG, van Beeck EF, Leenen LP. Long-term quality of life after surgical intensive care admission. *Arch Surg.* 2011;146(4): 412–418.

47. Hopkins RO, Weaver LK, Chan KJ, Orme JF, Jr. Quality of life, emotional, and cognitive function following acute respiratory distress syndrome. *J Int Neuropsychol Soc.* 2004;10(7):1005–1017.

48. Sukantarat KT, Burgess PW, Williamson RC, Brett SJ. Prolonged cognitive dysfunction in survivors of critical illness. *Anaesthesia.* 2005;60(9):847–853.

49. Rothenhausler HB, Ehrentraut S, Stoll C, Schelling G, Kapfhammer HP. The relationship between cognitive performance and employment and health status in long-term survivors of the acute respiratory distress syndrome: results of an exploratory study. *Gen Hosp Psychiatry.* 2001;23(2):88–94.

50. Ehlenbach WJ, Hough CL, Crane PK, et al. Association between acute care and critical illness hospitalization and cognitive function in older adults. *JAMA.* 2010;303(8):763–770.

51. Iwashyna TJ, Cooke CR, Wunsch H, Kahn JM. Population burden of long-term survivorship after severe sepsis in older Americans. *J Am Geriatr Soc.* 2012;60(6):1070–1077.

Psychological Impact of Critical Illness

O. JOSEPH BIENVENU AND CHRISTINA JONES

A few years back, Drs. Dale Needham and Joe Bienvenu spoke with a *New York Times* reporter, as Dale had begun a program to reduce sedation and start early physical therapy in the Johns Hopkins Medical Intensive Care Unit (ICU), and he had just published an article about this in *JAMA*.[1] Dale recommended that the journalist speak with this chapter's first author, who gave a quote or two about the frightening delirium-related experiences patients often have while critically ill and sedated. To our surprise, many people commented on the article, and others sent us emails, mostly about frightening psychotic experiences they had had while critically ill.

Here is an online comment:

I spent 10 days completely sedated on a ventilator in an ICU, suffering from respiratory failure/acute respiratory distress syndrome (ARDS). I had a 10-day-long hallucinative nightmare, which featured such things as my children dying, having a dead body next to me in bed, being naked in a truck stop, and more.

Here is a paraphrased email:

Last year I was hospitalized with severe pneumonia, and I spent a week in the ICU. I have never been so terrified. I was certain I had been abducted, locked in a torture chamber, and sexually assaulted. Later, on the hospital ward, I was noticeably frightened, and the doctors sent me for a brain scan because of my strange behavior. My husband took excellent care of me, in the hospital and at home afterwards, but he had no idea what I was talking about when I brought up my nightmarish experiences. In addition, the doctors and nurses couldn't explain it, and I felt confused and foolish. For a while, I also had trouble with routine things like completing the daily crossword puzzle, even using the telephone. Recently I've been having nightmares and flashbacks about the episode, around the 1-year anniversary of the incident. Your article helped me to understand what happened and may still be happening to me as a result of my illness and intensive care experience. It is a great relief to know that I am not alone, and not at fault.

These comments reflect frightening critical illness– and delirium-related persecutory experiences (which are often remembered quite vividly), as well as mild posttraumatic stress symptoms (the latter patient). As highlighted in Chapter 3, the latter patient had also had at least temporary cognitive impairment.

Over the years, we have had the opportunity to meet with many patients who have survived critical illnesses. The following example illustrates the suffering these patients face:

Mr. X is a single man in his 30s who was referred 6 months after his critical illness because of distressing recollections of his time in the ICU. He has a family history of affective disorder. He has felt vulnerable much of his life, and he attributes this to early-onset diabetes. Mr. X graduated from high school and took some college courses. He worked in his brother's business and made investments he later regretted due to his dislike of unpredictable drama. He dated in the past, never more than a month, and he has always lived with his parents. He quit smoking after his recent illness. He described himself as introverted and sensitive, and he had a pre–critical-illness history of substantial social anxiety, obsessive-compulsive, and depressive symptoms.

Mr. X was hospitalized for pneumonia complicated by sepsis, ARDS, and acute renal failure. He had to be intubated and treated with vasopressors, and he was in the hospital for about a month. After discharge, he recalled a number of awful experiences related to his ICU stay. Mr. X thought he had been kidnapped. He did not know where he was and tried to bite and kick the nurses, who he thought were torturing him. He remembered seeing children playing; when the children approached him, their faces were "blacked out." He saw blood and flesh coming out of the walls. Mr. X remained quite anxious and depressed much of the first 6 months after his critical illness. He had intrusive and distressing recollections of his ICU experience, and he avoided thinking and talking about it. He admitted feeling distant from others, and he felt unsafe. He was hypervigilant, his sleep was poor, and he had difficulty concentrating. Mr. X had substantial improvement in posttraumatic stress symptoms after his sertraline dose was increased.

Another example:

Mr. Y is a 39-year-old married man who was hospitalized for several weeks for treatment of pneumonia and ARDS, during which time he had agitated delirium (with frightening visual hallucinations and delusions that he was being genitally mutilated and killed). He was referred 6 months later because of flashbacks, avoidance/social withdrawal, hyperarousal symptoms, and a fear of recurrence of critical illness, with associated avoidance of and compulsive behavior related to germs. Mr. Y had also experienced physical weakness, demoralization, and problems with memory, attention, and executive functioning (e.g., losing keys and difficulty completing tasks, putting together furniture, and filling out a form for his son) since his critical illness.

Mr. Y had been a grocery store manager for 12 years prior to his critical illness, but he was laid off and replaced during his period of illness and recovery. Mr. Y has always been a hard worker who expects much of himself, so losing his job was quite difficult for him, and he was happy to get another, less demanding job. He and his wife of 4 years initially had difficulty after his illness because she didn't understand what he was going through and was embarrassed by his hypochondriasis.

Mr. Y went through a tremendous ordeal, facing many obstacles during and after his critical illness. His recovery was frustratingly slow at first, but he said meeting with a knowledgeable professional was helpful, as he realized he wasn't alone or unusual in experiencing the constellation of symptoms that are all too common in patients surviving critical illnesses.

Both of these cases illustrate posttraumatic stress phenomena, as well as the unique aspects of these phenomena, in critical illness survivors. That is, these patients are distressed in the context of having been on the verge of death, with life-saving medical procedures that are often not remembered as such. In addition, Mr. Y had had cognitive problems that seemed beyond those expected with hyperarousal alone.

In this chapter, we will explore the range of psychological distress phenomena experienced by critical illness survivors. The phenomena most commonly reported on are posttraumatic stress disorder (PTSD), depressive, and general (or nonspecific) anxiety symptoms, but it's important to note that patients also often have substantial bodily concerns and understandable worries about ever becoming ill again—particularly those with PTSD.[2]

WHAT IS STRESSFUL ABOUT CRITICAL ILLNESS
AND INTENSIVE CARE?

Patients with critical illnesses treated in ICUs face a number of severe psychic and physical stressors due to their illnesses, associated problems with physiology, and the procedures necessary to keep them alive. In particular, critically ill patients frequently experience:

1. Respiratory insufficiency, with low blood oxygen and elevated carbon dioxide levels, both of which are markedly anxiogenic. Note that having excessively low carbon dioxide can also be quite anxiogenic; this is an important balance.

2. Discomfort with endotracheal tube suctioning and invasive procedures. Having a tube in one's trachea is unnatural and can be quite uncomfortable, but this is only part of the stress related to intubation; endotracheal tubes must be suctioned deeply to prevent secretions from building up in the lungs, and deep suctioning is a markedly noxious experience. In addition, critically ill patients often need central intravenous lines placed, to draw blood, administer medications, and, sometimes, to monitor heart functioning. Also, some patients need tubes placed through their chest walls in order to drain fluid or air that accumulate and limit expansion of the lungs. Further, many patients require urinary bladder catheterization to prevent soiling and skin breakdown and monitor urine output. In addition, some patients similarly require rectal tubes to collect feces, especially liquid feces. Finally, most patients who are on mechanical ventilation need blood oxygenation monitoring via arterial lines. All of these procedures are painful, and if patients are not awake and aware of their purpose, it is not hard to see why patients remember being stabbed, sexually assaulted, tortured, and experimented upon.

3. Activation of the inflammatory cascade. Critical illnesses like sepsis typically involve massive inflammation throughout the body, damaging a number of organs, including the brain.

4. Strain on the hypothalamic–pituitary–adrenal axis. In the context of activation of the inflammatory cascade and leaking of blood vessels, the brain releases adrenocorticotropic hormone (ACTH) to stimulate release of cortisol from the cortices of the adrenal glands. However, the adrenal glands tend to be less responsive to ACTH in the context of massive inflammation, so cortisol levels can be lower than expected given high ACTH levels.

5. High levels of endogenous and exogenous catecholamines. Particularly in the absence of adequate endogenous cortisol levels, the adrenal medullae release norepinephrine and epinephrine to increase blood pressure. In addition, critical care clinicians provide exogenous catecholamines to maintain adequate blood pressure. It is important to keep in mind that catecholamines are considered stress mediators for a reason (discussed further later in the chapter).

6. Delirium with associated psychotic experiences. Though many critical care clinicians are aware of the importance of delirium, and some are now measuring this form of brain dysfunction, many clinicians do not appreciate the perceptual disturbances that can co-occur with delirium. As in the examples, patients have a very hard time discerning what is real from what is a nightmare-like distortion of reality, and persecutory delusions and visual hallucinations are common.

7. A limited ability to communicate. Patients with endotracheal tubes obviously can't speak, and excessive sedation (sometimes necessary to ensure adequate oxygenation), delirium, and/or muscle weakness can prevent patients from writing legibly. Patients with tracheostomies can sometimes

have speaking valves attached, but communication can
remain quite difficult.

8. Reduced autonomy. Critically ill patients are often entirely
   dependent on others—for survival, but also to address
   their basic needs. Their reduced ability to communicate
   complicates this reliance on others.

In addition, many survivors have cognitive and physical impairments
(including muscle weakness),[3–5] as well as financial strain, further hospitalization needs, and other stressors.[6,7] These stresses likely increase the
risk of psychiatric disturbances substantially.

POSTTRAUMATIC STRESS PHENOMENA—A BRIEF SUMMARY

Phenomenology

PTSD and related symptoms are perhaps the most vivid psychological
distress phenomena experienced by critical illness survivors. Survivors
often have intrusive memories and nightmares related to their critical illness and intensive care experiences, including fearing they will die, noxious physical stimuli, such as deep suctioning of endotracheal tubes, and
frightening hallucinations and paranoid delusional thoughts (e.g., that
staff are trying to kill them). Many critical illness survivors have difficulty
falling asleep, irritability, and poor concentration, and many try to avoid
hospitals, germs, or talking about their experiences.

Patients with post–critical illness PTSD often worry about becoming ill
again, and, as noted in the case of Mr. Y, they can go to great lengths to avoid
this. Some patients exhibit frank compulsions—for example, one of our
patients washed her whole body with an alcohol-based disinfectant in order
to prevent infection—but similar compulsions and/or avoidance are common. Substantial somatoform symptoms appear common in these patients.[2]

Prevalence

Several narrative and systematic reviews have addressed PTSD phenomena in critical illness survivors,[8–12] including a recent meta-analysis.[13] Though the prevalence of substantial PTSD symptoms or PTSD diagnoses varies by setting and assessment method, it appears that at least 20% of critical illness survivors are affected;[11,13] patients with ARDS and/or septic shock may have higher prevalences.[9–11,14] Importantly, PTSD phenomena are associated with worse quality of life and, in one study, a need for more frequent medical rehospitalizations.[10,11,13,15]

Risk Factors

PRE-ILLNESS RISK FACTORS

Risk factors for PTSD in critical illness survivors overlap, to some extent, with risk factors for PTSD in other settings.[16] For example, patients with a history of anxiety, depression, or other mental illness are at increased risk for PTSD when they experience critical illness and intensive care, and certain personality traits likely also increase risk.[11,13,14,17] Also, younger patients, women, and those less educated may be at increased risk.[11,13]

CRITICAL ILLNESS– AND INTENSIVE CARE–RELATED RISK FACTORS

Interestingly, severity of critical illness is *not* associated with later PTSD in survivors.[11,13] Neither is ICU length of stay,[11,13] except perhaps in ARDS survivors, for whom results are inconsistent.[10,14,18]

However, several indirect lines of evidence suggest that delirium increases risk for PTSD in survivors. First, agitation and need for physical restraint (markers of hyperactive delirium) are associated with later PTSD.[11] Second, high doses of benzodiazepines and opioids (which increase the risk of delirium) are associated with later PTSD.[11,13,14] Finally, early post-ICU memories of nightmarish psychotic experiences (e.g., frightening, vivid visual hallucinations and delusions of being imprisoned, tortured, sexually assaulted—evidence of having been delirious) are

associated with later PTSD.[11,13] Notably, a need for higher in-ICU sedative doses and later memories of frightening psychotic experiences appear
more common in patients with pre–critical illness histories of anxiety and
depression;[19] thus causal relationships are not straightforward.

As noted in Chapter 6, some in-ICU and post-ICU interventions appear
to reduce the risk of later PTSD. For example, in-ICU administration of
stress doses of corticosteroids and an in-ICU psychological intervention
appeared to reduce long-term PTSD risk, as did providing an ICU diary
to allow coherent processing of what occurred.[11,13,20]

POST–CRITICAL ILLNESS RISK FACTORS

Notably, psychological distress and less adaptive coping early in the recovery period are powerful predictors of later PTSD symptoms.[11,13] Figure 4.1
summarizes risk and protective factors and correlates of PTSD phenomena in survivors of critical illness.

POSTTRAUMATIC STRESS PHENOMENA—PERSONAL ACCOUNT

Background

In the mid-2000s, two critical care physicians, Drs. Peter Pronovost and
Dale Needham, approached me, this chapter's first author (OJB), to gauge
my interest in reviewing the literature on psychiatric distress phenomena
in critical illness survivors. I was very busy studying anxiety and depressive disorders in general population samples, particularly how these conditions were related to general personality traits, using longitudinal and
genetically informative data. So I wasn't particularly excited about this
new endeavor, even though I knew the two critical care specialists were
terrific researchers, clinicians, and people, and that increased my willing-
ness. I reluctantly said I would look for a fellow to help us with this project,
and I found Dr. Dimitry Davydow, who was looking for research projects
in the field of psychosomatic medicine (the interface of psychiatry with

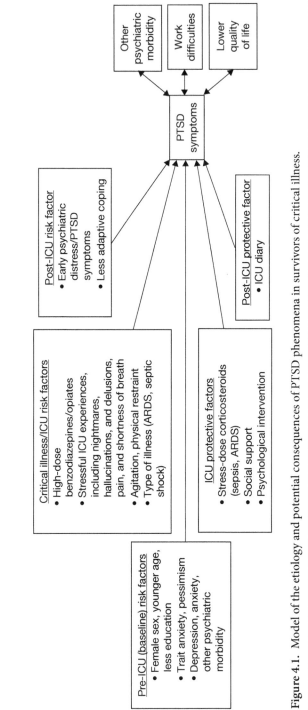

Figure 4.1. Model of the etiology and potential consequences of PTSD phenomena in survivors of critical illness.

the rest of medicine). We started working with Dale and a pulmonary/ critical care medicine fellow, Dr. Sanjay Desai (now residency director in internal medicine at Johns Hopkins Hospital), focusing initially on psychiatric morbidity in ARDS survivors. As we painstakingly combed the literature, we came across several rich and provocative articles by the second author of this chapter, Dr. Christina Jones, and we also started meeting with patients who were participating in an ARDS long-term outcomes study. The combination of research and clinical experiences with these patients drove Dimitry and me to delve deeper into this fascinating but understudied field.

PTSD phenomena in ARDS survivors

When we began combing the literature, it became clear that there were too many relevant studies to review systematically in a single manuscript. Since we had an ongoing study of ARDS (also known as "acute lung injury") survivors at the time,[21] and since we consider ARDS an "archetypal" critical illness,[22] we decided to start with ARDS and review all distress-related psychiatric outcomes.

In our post-ARDS psychiatric morbidity systematic review,[10] 10 observational studies met our inclusion criteria (total $n = 331$),[2,23–31] although not all of these studies had measures of PTSD. In this review, the point prevalence of clinically significant PTSD symptoms as ascertained via questionnaire ranged from 21% to 35%. Strikingly, the point prevalence of PTSD diagnosed by psychiatrists administering a structured interview ranged from 44% at hospital discharge to 24% at 8-year follow-up. A few risk factors for PTSD and/or PTSD symptoms were evident, including duration of sedation. We wondered whether sedation was meaningfully related to delirium, which in turn was a risk factor for PTSD, or whether patients at risk for PTSD because of in-ICU anxiety and agitation simply needed more sedatives, but we needed more information. In fact, we weren't even sure if duration of sedation was an important factor, as duration of sedation was very highly correlated with durations of mechanical ventilation and ICU stay.

PTSD phenomena in other critical illness survivors

With our interest piqued, we next decided to conduct a systematic review of PTSD and PTSD symptoms in general ICU survivors; we excluded studies focused on ARDS survivors (having reviewed these separately), as well as studies of survivors from specialty ICUs, such as cardiac care units or neurological and neurosurgical ICUs.[11] At the time (October of 2007), we identified 15 eligible articles, all about PTSD,[19,32–45] and with many more patients than in our post-ARDS psychiatric morbidity review (n = 1,104 who completed questionnaires, and n = 93 who had been interviewed by a clinician). The median study point prevalence of clinically significant symptoms of PTSD as ascertained via questionnaire was 22%, a bit lower than what we found in ARDS survivors but still quite high. Similarly, the median study point prevalence of doctoral-level clinician-diagnosed PTSD was 19%. But the most interesting part of this review was examining risk factors for post-ICU PTSD. We found that, as in most populations,[16] a potent predictor of post-ICU PTSD phenomena was prior psychiatric illness, including anxiety and depressive conditions; put another way, persons with prior psychiatric illness appear vulnerable to PTSD given the stress of critical illness. In addition, we reported research suggesting that stress doses of corticosteroids had a PTSD prevention effect. We also reported that, as we had suspected, in-ICU benzodiazepine administration was associated with PTSD symptoms, although we were not sure if or how benzodiazepine administration and PTSD were related causally. Finally, we reported that, as Jones first reported,[33] early post-ICU memories of frightening nightmares, hallucinations, and persecutory delusions were associated with later PTSD symptoms. We again wondered about the possible influence of delirium on PTSD phenomena, as benzodiazepines are deliriogenic, and delusions and hallucinations are common in delirium.

Recently, our group at Johns Hopkins conducted another systematic review of post-ICU PTSD, this time excluding studies of patients with particular critical illnesses and including a meta-analysis.[13] We found that the literature, beyond our own work,[14,46] had virtually exploded on this topic, so it was a good time to take another look. This time, we found 40 eligible papers on 36 unique cohorts (total $n = 4,260$).[17,19,32-41,43,47-73] We reported that, between 1 and 6 months after the ICU, the prevalence of clinically important PTSD symptoms was 25% to 44% (depending on the questionnaire score threshold), and, between 7 and 12 months after the ICU, the prevalence was between 17% and 34%; these prevalences were estimated using the most commonly administered PTSD symptom measure in this field,[74] the Impact of Event Scale (IES) questionnaire.[75] Again, ICU-related risk factors for post-ICU PTSD included benzodiazepine administration and early post-ICU memories of frightening ICU experiences. We also noted that the use of ICU diaries appeared to reduce the risk of PTSD in a European study conducted by Jones and her colleagues (to be discussed in Chapter 6).[47]

Does in-ICU delirium "cause" PTSD?

As noted, the evidence that delirium is causally related to post–critical illness PTSD is all indirect. That is, factors causally related to delirium are associated with PTSD (e.g., high-dose benzodiazepines and opiates), factors that reflect agitated delirium are associated with PTSD (e.g., need for physical restraints), and frightening memories of nightmares, persecutory delusions, and hallucinations while critically ill are strongly associated with later PTSD. But what about delirium measured as such? Interestingly, to our knowledge, no investigators have been able to link in-ICU delirium itself with PTSD, although several have addressed this issue.[14,19,39] In at least two of these studies,[14,39] delirium was virtually ubiquitous; that is, almost all of the critical illness survivors in these studies had been delirious at some point during their ICU stay. This is relevant because the investigators in both of the latter studies had to address the issue by attempting to relate *duration* of in-ICU delirium, rather than *presence* of in-ICU delirium, with later PTSD; no relationship with duration was evident. However, even if in-ICU delirium is not *causally* related to post-ICU PTSD, its presence *colors* the experience through memories of frightening experiences in the ICU.

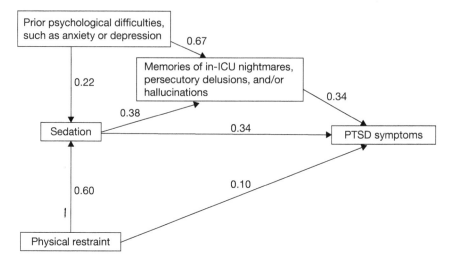

Figure 4.2. Path diagram of the factors associated with the development of PTSD symptoms in survivors of critical illness (adapted from Jones C, Bäckman C, Capuzzo M, et al., 2007).

A study by Jones and her colleagues delved into multiple relevant causal issues simultaneously, and the results were very interesting.[19] Briefly, Dr. Jones and her RACHEL group colleagues conducted a highly informative path analysis using data from a large multicenter European cohort of critical illness survivors followed longitudinally (see Figure 4.2). Several important conclusions can be drawn from this elegant study:

1. Prior psychological difficulties, such as anxiety and depression, predispose patients to frightening memories of in-ICU nightmares, persecutory delusions, and hallucinations in the context of critical illness.

2. Prior psychological difficulties predispose patients to higher sedative doses in the context of critical illness (i.e., these are *not* independent; patients with prior psychological difficulties presumably appear more distressed and are more agitated in the context of critical illness, and ICU clinicians respond with higher sedative doses to keep patients safe).

3. Needing physical restraint is also associated with higher sedative doses (presumably, patients' agitation and need for restraint prompts increased sedative doses, although the opposite is also possible; i.e., it is possible that the arrow here should be bidirectional).
4. Higher sedative doses predispose patients to frightening memories of in-ICU nightmares, persecutory delusions, and hallucinations.
5. Frightening memories of in-ICU nightmares, persecutory delusions, and hallucinations; higher sedative doses; and physical restraint independently increase risk for PTSD.

What was that about in-ICU corticosteroids reducing risk for PTSD after critical illness?

Reports that administering glucocorticoids could prevent PTSD after critical illness were counterintuitive to many of us. After all, these drugs are known to precipitate a variety of unwanted psychiatric phenomena, including delirium and mood disturbances (anxiety, mania, depression, and suicidal behavior).[76,77]

Potential PTSD preventive effects of glucocorticoids were first noted in survivors of septic shock in a case–control study.[45] Briefly, a group of German clinician investigators were simultaneously studying (1) the effects of stress doses of hydrocortisone on the hemodynamics of septic shock[78] and (2) PTSD after critical illness,[27] and they noticed that patients who had received stress-dose hydrocortisone had substantially less PTSD symptoms. They followed this case–control study with a small randomized controlled trial ($n = 20$) and reported that, in the group of patients who were randomized to stress-dose hydrocortisone, only 1 of 9 developed PTSD, compared to 7 of 11 patients randomized to placebo.[44] The same authors next tested the effects of perioperative low-dose hydrocortisone on PTSD after cardiac surgery in randomized controlled trials, and, though PTSD was not as common in this patient group, the authors again found a preventive effect.[79,80]

Observational studies have also addressed this issue. For example, Boer and colleagues followed a cohort of patients who had survived abdominal sepsis and reported that the number of days patients were administered hydrocortisone during the first 2 weeks of intensive care was unrelated to PTSD symptoms at follow-up.[81] However, in our longitudinal study in ARDS survivors, patients who received corticosteroids for larger proportions of their ICU stay had lower prevalences of clinically significant PTSD symptoms during 2-year follow-up.[14]

Why might patients administered stress doses of glucocorticoids be protected from PTSD? Several potential explanations may be applicable:[14,82]

1. Administering corticosteroids to patients with insufficient endogenous responses to adrenocorticotrophic hormone may result in less need for patients' bodies to respond with increased endogenous release of catecholamines (or, similarly, less need for clinicians to administer catecholamines to maintain adequate blood pressure).[80,82] Catecholamines are thought to activate the amygdala and enhance traumatic memory formation and fear conditioning.[83-85] Although catecholamines normally do not cross the blood–brain barrier, evidence from nonhuman animal models suggest that catecholamines do cross the blood–brain barrier when the latter becomes "leaky"[86,87]—for example, in sepsis.[88-90] But even if the blood–brain barrier is intact, peripheral catecholamines can affect the amygdala and enhance traumatic memory formation and fear conditioning indirectly through the vagus nerve.[91]

2. Corticosteroids can also have direct effects on memory formation and retrieval.[82] For example, low serum cortisol in patients critically ill with ARDS has been associated with more memories of traumatic experiences during the critical illness.[92] However, studies of the preventive effect of stress-dose hydrocortisone administration do not suggest that replenishing glucocorticoids reduces the risk of PTSD by

affecting recall of traumatic experiences.[44,79,80] It is possible
that exogenous hydrocortisone given during critical illness
has a salutary effect on the salience of these memories, but
this remains unclear.

3. One possibility, studied only a little thus far,[80] is that
corticosteroids reduce inflammation during critical illness,
and this reduction in inflammation is responsible for
glucocorticoids' salutary effect in preventing PTSD and,
possibly, other distress-related psychiatric conditions.[11,93]

Regardless of the possible mechanism(s) by which in-ICU corticosteroids
may prevent PTSD in survivors of critical illness, to our knowledge no
clinicians routinely administer corticosteroids for this purpose. That is,
this is not part of typical critical care medicine practice.

What about measurement of PTSD phenomena?

As noted, most studies of critical illness survivors have employed questionnaire measures, with thresholds for clinically significant PTSD symptoms. That is, most studies have not used clinicians to perform structured
or semi-structured psychiatric interviews with the patients. A reasonable
question is how well questionnaires perform versus more rigorous diagnostic assessments.

To our knowledge, the first clinical psychometric validation study of a
PTSD assessment tool in survivors of critical illness compared results of
a modified version of the Post-Traumatic Stress Syndrome 10-Questions
Inventory (PTSS-10)[94–96] to psychiatrists' diagnoses of PTSD using the
Structured Clinical Interview for DSM-IV (SCID-IV)[97] in survivors of
ARDS.[28] The authors modified the PTSS-10 in two ways. First, they added
questions regarding memories of the patient's time in the ICU, specifically
regarding nightmares, severe anxiety or panic, severe pain, and short-
ness of breath or feelings of suffocation; they call this section Part A of
the modified questionnaire. Notably, Part A covers both accurate real-life

experiences of critical illness (i.e., pain, fear, and dyspnea), as well as one of those other frightening experiences during critical illness, nightmares. Part B of the modified instrument is similar to the original version of the PTSS-10, which covers sleep disturbance, nightmares, depression, hyperalertness, emotional and social withdrawal (emotional numbing and inability to care for others), irritability, moodiness, guilt, avoidance of reminders of the trauma, and muscle tension. The authors changed the wording of the ninth item to be more directly relevant to a patient's ICU experience ("fear of places and situations which remind me of the intensive care unit"). Each of the 10 items is rated on a seven-point scale, reflecting symptom frequency; the potential total score ranges from 10 to 70. As the authors noted, the original PTSS-10 was based on an earlier conception of PTSD,[98] and some of the items are less relevant to a more modern conception of PTSD (e.g., depressed mood, muscle tension).[99] Nevertheless, this modified form of the PTSS-10 performed well psychometrically, with high internal consistency (Cronbach's α = 0.89), test-retest reliability (intraclass correlation coefficient α = 0.89), and construct validity (a monotonic relationship between the number of Part A "traumatic memories" and Part B scores, Spearman's ρ = 0.48). In addition, the authors demonstrated high criterion validity of the Part B score versus psychiatrist's diagnoses of DSM-IV PTSD, with a sensitivity of 77% and specificity of 98% at a cut-off value of 35.

Later, Twigg and colleagues (including Dr. Jones) expanded the PTSS-10 to create the PTSS-14,[62] since the PTSS-10 focused mostly on hyperarousal symptoms (five items), with only one item addressing re-experiencing or intrusion phenomena (i.e., nightmares) and one item addressing avoidance and numbing (withdrawal from others). The PTSS-14 adds another intrusion item ("Upsetting, unwanted thoughts or images of my time on the intensive care unit"), as well as an additional avoidance item ("Avoid places, people or situations that remind me of the intensive care unit") and two "numbness" items ("Feeling numb [e.g., cannot cry, unable to have loving feelings]" and "Feeling as if my plans or dreams of the future will not come true"). Each of the 14 items is rated on a seven-point scale, reflecting symptom frequency; the potential total score ranges from 14 to

98. The authors validated the PTSS-14 against a previously validated diagnostic questionnaire, the Posttraumatic Stress Diagnostic Scale (PDS).[100] The authors reported high internal consistency (α ranged between 0.84 and 0.89), high test-retest reliability (intraclass correlation coefficient as high as 0.90), high concurrent validity (Pearson's r as high as 0.86 with the PDS symptom severity score and as high as 0.71 with the IES total score), and high predictive validity (Pearson's r as high as 0.85 with the PDS symptom severity score and as high as 0.71 with the IES total score). A receiver operating curve (ROC) analysis indicated very good sensitivity (as high as 86%) and specificity (as high as 97%) at a cut-off value of 45. The area under the ROC curve (AUC) ranged from 82% to 95%.

Most recently, Bienvenu and colleagues validated the revised version of the IES, the IES-R,[101] against the current gold standard structured clinical interview for PTSD, the Clinician-Administered PTSD Scale (CAPS),[102] in ARDS survivors.[99] The IES-R is a 22-item questionnaire; each item is rated on a five-point severity scale. The developers recommend using a mean score for either the total score or for subscale scores (in either case, the potential mean score range is between 0 and 4). The internal consistency of the IES-R was high in the study (α = 0.96). The IES-R total score (actual range 0.0 to 3.2) and CAPS total severity score (actual range 0–70) were strongly correlated (Pearson's r = 0.80; Spearman's ρ = 0.69). Using CAPS data, 13% of the survivors had PTSD at the time of assessment, and 27% had at least partial PTSD. In an ROC curve analysis with CAPS PTSD or partial PTSD as criterion variables, the AUC ranged from 95% to 97%. At an IES-R threshold (total mean score) of 1.6, with the same criterion variables, sensitivities ranged from 80% to 100%, specificities 85% to 91%, positive predictive values 50% to 75%, negative predictive values 93% to 100%, positive likelihood ratios 6.5 to 9.0, negative likelihood ratios 0.0 to 0.2, and efficiencies 87% to 90%. We concluded that the IES-R is an excellent brief symptom measure and screening tool for PTSD in ARDS survivors.

To our knowledge, no one has assessed the psychometric properties of a screening instrument for PTSD in critical illness survivors against the new gold standard set with the publication of the fifth edition of the *Diagnostic and Statistical Manual of Mental Disorders.*[103,104] Nevertheless, we feel that, for now, the PTSS-14 and IES-R are reasonable measures and that these measures are aimed at the same core construct.[105]

DEPRESSIVE PHENOMENA

Phenomenology

Depressive phenomena have also received substantial attention in the critical illness outcomes literature; depressive mood states are relatively common in survivors.[106,107] Loss of energy, poor concentration, and sleep difficulties are particularly common in this population; many patients also report low mood and anhedonia (loss of interest and pleasure).

Prevalence

Although the prevalence of depressive symptoms or depression-related diagnoses varies by setting and assessment method, it appears that about 30% of critical illness survivors are affected.[106,107] Importantly, depressive phenomena in critical illness survivors are associated with worse quality of life and impaired physical function.[106,108]

Risk Factors

PRE-ILLNESS RISK FACTORS

Risk factors for depressed mood in survivors of critical illness overlap to some extent with risk factors for depression in other settings. For example, patients with a history of depression or other mental illness are at increased risk for depressive mood states given critical illness and intensive care.[106,107,109] Also, women, those less educated, and underemployed people may be at increased risk.[106,108,109]

CRITICAL ILLNESS– AND INTENSIVE CARE–RELATED RISK FACTORS

As with PTSD, severity of critical illness is *not* associated with later depressive symptoms in survivors; neither is ICU length of stay.[106,107]

Although studied less frequently than in PTSD, early memories of nightmares, persecutory hallucinations, and delusions have been associated with later depressive phenomena in survivors.[107]

As noted in Chapter 6, an in-ICU psychological intervention appeared effective in reducing depressive and other psychological distress symptoms in survivors.[20]

POST–CRITICAL ILLNESS RISK FACTORS

Notably, psychological distress (including, but not limited to, depressive symptoms) and less adaptive coping early in the recovery period are powerful predictors of later depressive symptoms, and depressive phenomena tend to co-occur with other psychiatric distress phenomena.[46,106,107] Figure 4.3 presents a model of the etiology and potential consequences of depressive phenomena in survivors of critical illness.

DEPRESSIVE PHENOMENA—SOME MORE DETAIL

As with PTSD, our group at Johns Hopkins first systematically reviewed depressive symptoms in ARDS survivors.[10] Also as with PTSD, our research group at Johns Hopkins has conducted two systematic reviews of clinically significant depressive symptoms and depressive disorders in patients who have experienced critical illness and intensive care; the more recent review included a meta-analysis.[106,107]

In our post-ARDS psychiatric morbidity systematic review,[10] the point prevalence of clinically significant depressive symptoms as ascertained via questionnaire ranged from 17% to 43%. However, only one study used clinicians to assess patients using a structured interview; at a median of 8 years after ARDS, the prevalence of major depressive disorder was 4% (similar to the general population prevalence in German adults at the time).[2]

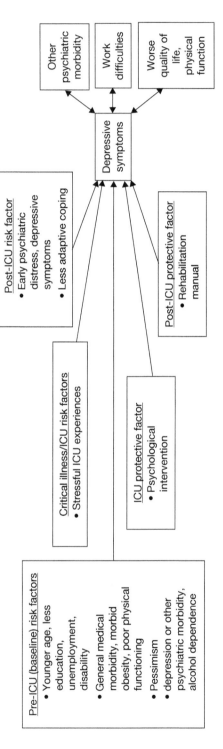

Figure 4.3. Model of the etiology and potential consequences of depressive phenomena in survivors of critical illness.

In our first systematic review of depressive symptoms and disorders, we focused on general ICU survivors; we excluded studies focused on ARDS survivors (having reviewed these separately), as well as studies of survivors from specialty ICUs, such as cardiac care units or neurological and neurosurgical ICUs.[106] At the time (October of 2007), we identified 14 eligible articles, all about depressive phenomena,[33,34,36,37,41-43,110-116] and with many more patients than in our post-ARDS psychiatric morbidity review (n = 1,213 who completed questionnaires, 134 of whom had been interviewed by a clinician). The median study point prevalence of clinically significant depressive symptoms as ascertained via questionnaire was 28%. Similarly, the single study point prevalence of clinician-diagnosed depressive disorders at 2-month follow-up was 33%; although slightly less than half of these patients were assessed as being in the midst of a major depressive episode, 49% of the patients were on an antidepressant (more than half of whom had not been on an antidepressant prior to the index critical illness).[113]

In our more recent systematic review and meta-analysis, we found 42 eligible papers reporting on 38 unique cohorts (total n = 4,113).[17,33,34,36,37,41-43,48,50-56,59,61,65,107,110,111,113,115,117-134] We reported that the prevalence of clinically important depressive symptoms was 29% between 2 and 3 months after the critical illness, 34% 6 months after the critical illness, and 29% 12 to 14 months after the critical illness. These prevalences were estimated using the most commonly administered depression symptom measure in this field,[74] the Hospital Anxiety and Depression Scale (HADS) questionnaire (depression subscale),[135] although the prevalences were comparable when we included other measures.

While the HADS has been validated in a number of medically ill and other populations,[136] it has not been validated against a gold standard structured or semi-structured diagnostic interview specifically in critical illness survivors. An advantage, though, of the HADS is that it de-emphasizes symptoms of general medical illness like loss of appetite and low energy, unlike some other measures.[137]

We recently performed a limited psychometric evaluation of the HADS administered in the context of a longitudinal cohort study of ARDS survivors.[138] Internal consistency of the anxiety and depression subscales was good ($\alpha \geq 0.7$), and exploratory factor analysis suggested the familiar two-factor structure found in most populations. In addition, the anxiety and depression subscales were correlated with mental health quality of life measures, evidence of convergent validity.[138]

A NOTE ABOUT GENERAL OR NONSPECIFIC ANXIETY PHENOMENA

Our group at Johns Hopkins first systematically reviewed general or non-specific anxiety symptoms in ARDS survivors.[10] In this review, the point prevalence of clinically significant anxiety symptoms as ascertained via questionnaire ranged from 17% to 43%. However, none of the studies used clinicians to assess patients via a structured interview.

Later, we conducted two studies of general anxiety symptoms (as assessed using the HADS anxiety subscale) in ARDS survivors. In the first study, the prevalence of suprathreshold general anxiety symptoms was 38% at 3-month follow-up, and correlates included prior psychiatric morbidity and elevated body mass index, as well as more dependencies in instrumental activities of daily living and worse health-related quality of life at follow-up.[139] In the second study, the prevalence of suprathreshold general anxiety symptoms at 6- and 12-month follow-up was similar, ~42%.[18] We noted high comorbidity with suprathreshold symptoms of depression and PTSD, as well as significant associations with several baseline factors (younger age, female sex, unemployment, alcohol misuse) and one ICU factor (greater opioid use). Again, severity of illness and ICU length of stay were unrelated to general anxiety symptoms.[18]

Recently, we conducted a systematic review and meta-analysis of general or nonspecific anxiety phenomena in survivors of critical illness.[140] We found 27 eligible unique patient cohorts (total n = 2,880).[17,33,34,36,37,41–43,48,50,52-54,56,61,65,115,119–120,123–126,129–131] We reported that the prevalence of clinically important depressive symptoms was 32% between 2 and 3 months after the critical illness, 40% 6 months after the critical illness, and 34% 12 to 14 months after the critical illness. These prevalences were estimated using the most commonly administered anxiety measure in this field, the HADS questionnaire (anxiety subscale).[135] As with depressive phenomena, anxiety symptoms were more common in patients who had psychiatric distress during the index admission, as well as in those who remembered frightening nightmares, persecutory delusions, and hallucinations during the ICU stay. Physical rehabilitation and ICU diaries showed potential benefit for post-ICU anxiety symptoms.[140]

To date, the nature of these general or nonspecific anxiety phenomena remains unclear. For example, we are unsure whether these reflect post-traumatic stress, illness anxiety, or other symptoms. This is an important question for future studies.

DO CRITICAL ILLNESS AND INTENSIVE CARE "CAUSE" PSYCHIATRIC DISORDERS?

Some may wonder whether the immense stress of critical illness and intensive care is actually relevant to the development or worsening of mental distress, or whether psychiatric morbidity is simply constant before and after critical illness. Several studies have addressed this issue, using data collected before and after critical illness and intensive care:[46]

1. Dimitry Davydow and colleagues at the University of Washington examined data from a longitudinal study of patients with diabetes, the Pathways Epidemiologic Follow-up Study.[134,141] In the first study, the authors noted that patients who had a critical illness and ICU stay were at increased risk for clinically significant depressive symptoms at follow-up.[141] Interestingly, in the second study, the authors established that the opposite was also true. That is, patients with clinically significant depressive symptoms were also at increased risk for critical illness requiring intensive care.[134] These results suggest bidirectional longitudinal relationships

between critical illness/intensive care and psychiatric
morbidity; they do *not* suggest constancy of psychiatric
phenomena.

2. In another study, Dr. Davydow and colleagues examined data
    from the Health and Retirement Study, a population-based
    longitudinal cohort study of older adults.[142] In that study, the
    authors found that the prevalence of clinically significant
    depressive symptoms remained constant approximately
    a year before and a year after an episode of severe sepsis.
    Unlike the prior studies, this study suggested that, in older
    adults, severe sepsis surprisingly did not increase the risk of
    clinically significant depression.[142] This study is an outlier.

3. In the most recent study we are aware of on this issue, Wunsch
    and colleagues examined linked data from longitudinal
    medical databases in the country of Denmark.[143] This is, by
    far, the largest study of its kind, including more than 24,000
    patients who were critically ill and required mechanical
    ventilation, as well as two matched comparison cohorts—
    non-critically ill hospitalized patients and the general
    population. The results were striking. Briefly, patients with
    a critical illness requiring mechanical ventilation were
    slightly more likely to have had a psychiatric diagnosis
    in the 5 years prior to the hospitalization than patients
    who were hospitalized but did not need intensive care
    (prevalence ratio 1.3). Also, patients with a critical illness
    requiring mechanical ventilation were substantially more
    likely to have had a psychiatric diagnosis in the
    5 years prior to the hospitalization than persons in
    the matched general population cohort (prevalence
    ratio 2.6). Also, patients who were hospitalized, whether or
    not they required intensive care, were more likely
    to be prescribed psychoactive medications than
    persons in the matched general population cohort

(prevalence ratio 1.4). However, after a hospitalization, critically ill patients requiring mechanical ventilation were substantially more likely to receive a new psychiatric diagnosis than patients who were hospitalized but did not require intensive care (adjusted hazard ratio 3.4) or persons in the general population (hazard ratio 22!). In addition, critically ill patients requiring mechanical ventilation were substantially more likely to be prescribed a psychoactive medication than patients who were hospitalized but did not require intensive care (adjusted hazard ratio 2.4) or persons in the general population (hazard ratio 21!). To summarize this important study,[143] the authors found that being diagnosed with a psychiatric illness and being prescribed a psychoactive medication were associated with a moderately increased risk for hospitalization. However, being hospitalized, *especially* with a critical illness, was associated with a markedly increased risk for receiving a new psychiatric diagnosis and/or a prescription for a psychoactive medication.

Weighing these results together, we opine that critical illness and intensive care quite substantially increase risk for psychiatric morbidity. Thus, it is unconscionable to consider not addressing these survivor's mental health needs.

CONCLUSIONS

Substantial PTSD, depressive, and general or nonspecific anxiety phenomena are common in critical illness survivors, and these phenomena are associated with diminished quality of life and functioning. In the next two chapters (Chapters 5 and 6), we will explore the growing literature on prevention of, and early intervention in, these syndromes.

REFERENCES

1. Needham DM. Mobilizing patients in the intensive care unit: improving neuro-muscular weakness and physical function. *JAMA*. 2008;300(14):1685–1690.
2. Kapfhammer HP, Rothenhäusler HB, Krauseneck T, et al. Posttraumatic stress disorder and health-related quality of life in long-term survivors of acute respiratory distress syndrome. *Am J Psychiatry*. 2004;161(1):45–52.
3. Herridge MS, Cheung AM, Tansey CM, et al. One-year outcomes in survivors of the acute respiratory distress syndrome. *N Engl J Med*. 2003;348(8):683–693.
4. Herridge MS, Tansey CM, Matté A, et al. Functional disability 5 years after acute respiratory distress syndrome. *N Engl J Med*. 2011;364(14):1293–1304.
5. Needham DM, Davidson J, Cohen H, et al. Improving long-term outcomes after discharge from intensive care unit: report from a stakeholders' conference. *Crit Care Med*. 2012;40(2):502–509.
6. Cheung AM, Tansey CM, Tomlinson G, et al. Two-year outcomes, health care use, and costs of survivors of acute respiratory distress syndrome. *Am J Respir Crit Care Med*. 2006;174(5):538–544.
7. Unroe M, Kahn JM, Carson SS, et al. One-year trajectories of care and resource utilization for recipients of prolonged mechanical ventilation: a cohort study. *Ann Intern Med*. 2010;153(3):167–175.
8. Jackson JC, Hart RP, Gordon SM, et al. Post-traumatic stress disorder and post-traumatic stress symptoms following critical illness in medical intensive care unit patients: assessing the magnitude of the problem. *Crit Care*. 2007;11(1):R27.
9. Griffiths J, Fortune G, Barber V, et al. The prevalence of posttraumatic stress disorder in survivors of ICU treatment: a systematic review. *Intensive Care Med*. 2007;33(9):1506–1518.
10. Davydow DS, Desai SV, Needham DM, et al. Psychiatric morbidity in survivors of the acute respiratory distress syndrome: a systematic review. *Psychosom Med*. 2008;70(4):512–519.
11. Davydow DS, Gifford JM, Desai SV, et al. Posttraumatic stress disorder in general intensive care unit survivors: a systematic review. *Gen Hosp Psychiatry*. 2008;30(5):421–434.
12. Wade D, Hardy R, Howell D, et al. Identifying clinical and acute psychological risk factors for PTSD after critical care: a systematic review. *Minerva Anestesiol*. 2013;79(8):944–963.
13. Parker AM, Sricharoenchai T, Raparla S, et al. Posttraumatic stress disorder in critical illness survivors: a metaanalysis. *Crit Care Med*. 2015;43(5):1121–1129.
14. Bienvenu OJ, Gellar J, Althouse BM, et al. Post-traumatic stress disorder symptoms after acute lung injury: a 2-year prospective longitudinal study. *Psychol Med*. 2013;43(12):2657–2671.
15. Davydow DS, Hough CL, Zatzick D, et al. Psychiatric symptoms and acute care service utilization over the course of the year following medical-surgical ICU admission: a longitudinal investigation. *Crit Care Med*. 2014;42(12):2473–2481.

16. Brewin CR, Andrews B, Valentine JD. Meta-analysis of risk factors for post-traumatic stress disorder in trauma-exposed adults. *J Consult Clin Psychol.* 2000;68(5):748–766.

17. Myhren H, Ekeberg O, Tøien K, et al. Posttraumatic stress, anxiety and depression symptoms in patients during the first year post intensive care unit discharge. *Crit Care.* 2010;14(1):R14.

18. Huang M, Parker AM, Bienvenu OJ, et al. Psychiatric symptoms in acute respiratory distress syndrome survivors: a 1-year national multicenter study. *Crit Care Med.* 2016;44(5):954–965.

19. Jones C, Bäckman C, Capuzzo M, et al. Precipitants of post-traumatic stress disorder following intensive care: a hypothesis generating study of diversity in care. *Intensive Care Med.* 2007;33(6):978–985.

20. Peris A, Bonizzoli M, Iozzelli D, et al. Early intra-intensive care unit psychological intervention promotes recovery from post traumatic stress disorders, anxiety and depression symptoms in critically ill patients. *Crit Care.* 2011;15(1):R41.

21. Needham DM, Dennison CR, Dowdy DW, et al. Study protocol: the Improving Care of Acute Lung Injury Patients (ICAP) study. *Crit Care.* 2006;10(1):R9.

22. Herridge MS, Angus DC. Acute lung injury—affecting many lives. *N Engl J Med.* 2005;353(16):1736–1738.

23. Hopkins RO, Weaver LK, Chan KJ, et al. Quality of life, cognitive, and emotional function following acute respiratory distress syndrome. *J Int Neuropsychol Soc.* 2004;10(7):1005–1017.

24. Shaw RJ, Harvey JE, Nelson KL, et al. Linguistic analysis to assess medically related posttraumatic stress symptoms. *Psychosomatics.* 2001;42(1):35–40.

25. Weinert CR, Gross CR, Kangas JR, et al. Health-related quality of life after acute lung injury. *Am J Respir Crit Care Med.* 1997;156(4 Pt 1):1120–1128.

26. Nelson BJ, Weinert CR, Bury CL, et al. Intensive care unit drug use and subsequent quality of life in acute lung injury patients. *Crit Care Med.* 2000;28(11):3626–3630.

27. Schelling G, Stoll C, Haller M, et al. Health-related quality of life and posttraumatic stress disorder in survivors of the acute respiratory distress syndrome. *Crit Care Med.* 1998;26(4):651–659.

28. Stoll C, Kapfhammer HP, Rothenhäusler HB, et al. Sensitivity and specificity of a screening test to document traumatic experiences and to diagnose post-traumatic stress disorder in ARDS patients after intensive care treatment. *Intensive Care Med.* 1999;25(7):697–704.

29. Hopkins RO, Weaver LK, Collingridge D, et al. Two-year cognitive, emotional, and quality-of-life outcomes in acute respiratory distress syndrome. *Am J Respir Crit Care Med.* 2005;171(4):340–347.

30. Christie JD, Biester RC, Taichman DB, et al. Formation and validation of a telephone battery to assess cognitive function in acute respiratory distress syndrome survivors. *J Crit Care.* 2006;21(2):125–132.

31. Deja M, Denke C, Weber-Carstens S, et al. Social support during intensive care unit stay might improve mental impairment and consequently health-related

quality of life in survivors of severe acute respiratory distress syndrome. *Crit Care.* 2006;10(5):R147.

32. Perrins J, King N, Collings J. Assessment of long-term psychological well-being following intensive care. *Intensive Crit Care Nurs.* 1998;14(3):108–116.

33. Jones C, Griffiths RD, Humphris G, et al. Memory, delusions, and the development of acute posttraumatic stress disorder-related symptoms after intensive care. *Crit Care Med.* 2001;29(3):573–580.

34. Samuelson KA, Lundberg D, Fridlund B. Stressful memories and psychological distress in adult mechanically ventilated intensive care patients: a 2-month follow-up study. *Acta Anaesthesiol Scand.* 2007;51(6):671–678.

35. Cuthbertson BH, Hull A, Strachan M, et al. Post-traumatic stress disorder after critical illness requiring general intensive care. *Intensive Care Med.* 2004;30(3):450–455.

36. Jones C, Skirrow P, Griffiths RD, et al. Rehabilitation after critical illness: a randomized, controlled trial. *Crit Care Med.* 2003;31(10):2456–2461.

37. Sukantarat K, Greer S, Brett S, et al. Physical and psychological sequelae of critical illness. *Br J Health Psychol.* 2007;12(Pt 1):65–74.

38. Griffiths J, Gager M, Alder N, et al. A self-report-based study of the incidence and associations of sexual dysfunction in survivors of intensive care treatment. *Intensive Care Med.* 2006;32(3):445–451.

39. Girard TD, Shintani AK, Jackson JC, et al. Risk factors for post-traumatic stress disorder symptoms following critical illness requiring mechanical ventilation: a prospective cohort study. *Crit Care.* 2007;11(1):R28.

40. Nickel M, Leiberich P, Nickel C, et al. The occurrence of posttraumatic stress disorder in patients following intensive care treatment: a cross-sectional study in a random sample. *J Intensive Care Med.* 2004;19(5):285–290.

41. Rattray JE, Johnston M, Wildsmith JA. Predictors of emotional outcomes of intensive care. *Anaesthesia.* 2005;60(11):1085–1092.

42. Kress JP, Gehlbach B, Lacy M, et al. The long-term psychological effects of daily sedative interruption on critically ill patients. *Am J Respir Crit Care Med.* 2003;168(12):1457–1461.

43. Scragg P, Jones A, Fauvel N. Psychological problems following ICU treatment. *Anaesthesia.* 2001;56(1):9–14.

44. Schelling G, Briegel J, Roozendaal B, et al. The effect of stress doses of hydrocortisone during septic shock on posttraumatic stress disorder in survivors. *Biol Psychiatry.* 2001;50(12):978–985.

45. Schelling G, Stoll C, Kapfhammer HP, et al. The effect of stress doses of hydrocortisone during septic shock on posttraumatic stress disorder and health-related quality of life in survivors. *Crit Care Med.* 1999;27(12):2678–2683.

46. Bienvenu OJ, Colantuoni E, Mendez-Tellez PA, et al. Cooccurrence of and remission from general anxiety, depression, and posttraumatic stress disorder symptoms after acute lung injury: a 2-year longitudinal study. *Crit Care Med.* 2015;43(3):642–653.

47. Jones C, Bäckman C, Capuzzo M, et al. Intensive care diaries reduce new-onset post-traumatic stress disorder following critical illness. *Crit Care.* 2010;14(5):R168.

48. Garrouste-Orgeas M, Coquet I, Périer A, et al. Impact of an intensive care unit diary on psychological distress in patients and relatives. *Crit Care Med.* 2012;40(7):2033–2040.

49. Sackey PV, Martling CR, Carlswärd C, et al. Short- and long-term follow-up of intensive care unit patients after sedation with isoflurane and midazolam—a pilot study. *Crit Care Med.* 2008;36(3):801–806.

50. Strøm T, Stylsvig M, Toft P. Long-term psychological effects of a no-sedation protocol in critically ill patients. *Crit Care.* 2011;15(6):R293.

51. Jackson JC, Girard TD, Gordon SM, et al. Long-term cognitive and psychological outcomes in the awakening and breathing controlled trial. *Am J Respir Crit Care Med.* 2010;182(2):183–191.

52. Treggiari MM, Romand JA, Yanez ND, et al. Randomized trial of light versus deep sedation on mental health after critical illness. *Crit Care Med.* 2009;37(9):2527–2534.

53. Cuthbertson BH, Rattray J, Campbell MK, et al. The PRaCTICaL study of nurse led, intensive care follow-up programmes for improving long-term outcomes from critical illness: a pragmatic randomised controlled trial. *BMJ.* 2009;339:b3723.

54. van der Schaaf M, Beelen A, Dongelmans DA, et al. Functional status after intensive care: a challenge for rehabilitation professionals to improve outcome. *J Rehabil Med.* 2009;41(5):360–366.

55. Paparrigopoulos T, Melissaki A, Tzavellas E, et al. Increased co-morbidity of depression and post-traumatic stress disorder symptoms and common risk factors in intensive care unit survivors: a two-year follow-up study. *Int J Psychiatry Clin Pract.* 2014;18(1):25–31.

56. Wade DM, Howell DC, Weinman JA, et al. Investigating risk factors for psychological morbidity three months after intensive care: a prospective cohort study. *Crit Care.* 2012;16(5):R192.

57. Azoulay E, Kouatchet A, Jaber S, et al. Noninvasive mechanical ventilation in patients having declined tracheal intubation. *Intensive Care Med.* 2013;39(2):292–301.

58. Davydow DS, Kohen R, Hough CL, et al. A pilot investigation of the association of genetic polymorphisms regulating corticotrophin-releasing hormone with post-traumatic stress and depressive symptoms in medical-surgical intensive care unit survivors. *J Crit Care.* 2014;29(1):101–106.

59. Davydow DS, Zatzick D, Hough CL, et al. A longitudinal investigation of post-traumatic stress and depressive symptoms over the course of the year following medical-surgical intensive care unit admission. *Gen Hosp Psychiatry.* 2013;35(3):226–232.

60. Bugedo G, Tobar E, Aguirre M, et al. The implementation of an analgesia-based sedation protocol reduced deep sedation and proved to be safe and feasible in patients on mechanical ventilation. *Rev Bras Ter Intensiva.* 2013;25(3):188–196.

61. Schandl A, Bottai M, Hellgren E, et al. Gender differences in psychological morbidity and treatment in intensive care survivors—a cohort study. *Crit Care.* 2012;16(3):R80.

62. Twigg E, Humphris G, Jones C, et al. Use of a screening questionnaire for post-traumatic stress disorder (PTSD) on a sample of UK ICU patients. *Acta Anaesthesiol Scand.* 2008;52(2):202–208.

63. Wallen K, Chaboyer W, Thalib L, et al. Symptoms of acute posttraumatic stress disorder after intensive care. *Am J Crit Care.* 2008;17(6):534–543.
64. Myhren H, Ekeberg Ø, Stokland O. Health-related quality of life and return to work after critical illness in general intensive care unit patients: a 1-year follow-up study. *Crit Care Med.* 2010;38(7):1554–1561.
65. Myhren H, Tøien K, Ekeberg O, et al. Patients' memory and psychological distress after ICU stay compared with expectations of the relatives. *Intensive Care Med.* 2009;35(12):2078–2086.
66. Weinert CR, Sprenkle M. Post-ICU consequences of patient wakefulness and sedative exposure during mechanical ventilation. *Intensive Care Med.* 2008; 34(1):82–90.
67. da Costa JB, Marcon SS, Rossi RM. Posttraumatic stress disorder and the presence of recollections from an intensive care unit stay. *J Brasil Psiquiatr.* 2012;61(1):13–19.
68. Schandl AR, Brattström OR, Svensson-Raskh A, et al. Screening and treatment of problems after intensive care: a descriptive study of multidisciplinary follow-up. *Intensive Crit Care Nurs.* 2011;27(2):94–101.
69. Granja C, Gomes E, Amaro A, et al. Understanding posttraumatic stress disorder-related symptoms after critical care: the early illness amnesia hypothesis. *Crit Care Med.* 2008;36(10):2801–2809.
70. Badia-Castelló M, Trujillano-Cabello J, Serviá-Goixart L, et al. Recall and memory after intensive care unit stay. Development of posttraumatic stress disorder. *Med Clin (Barc).* 2006;126(15):561–566.
71. Richter JC, Waydhas C, Pajonk FG. Incidence of posttraumatic stress disorder after prolonged surgical intensive care unit treatment. *Psychosomatics.* 2006;47(3):223–230.
72. Rattray J, Johnston M, Wildsmith JA. The intensive care experience: development of the ICE questionnaire. *J Adv Nurs.* 2004;47(1):64–73.
73. Van Ness PH, Murphy TE, Araujo KL, et al. Multivariate graphical methods provide an insightful way to formulate explanatory hypotheses from limited categorical data. *J Clin Epidemiol.* 2012;65(2):179–188.
74. Turnbull AE, Rabiee A, Davis WE, et al. Outcome measurement in ICU survivorship research from 1970 to 2013: a scoping review of 425 publications. *Crit Care Med.* 2016;44(7):1267–1277.
75. Horowitz M, Wilner N, Alvarez W. Impact of Event Scale: a measure of subjective stress. *Psychosom Med.* 1979;41(3):209–218.
76. Fardet L, Petersen I, Nazareth I. Suicidal behavior and severe neuropsychiatric disorders following glucocorticoid therapy in primary care. *Am J Psychiatry.* 2012;169(5):491–497.
77. Schreiber MP, Colantuoni E, Bienvenu OJ, et al. Corticosteroids and transition to delirium in patients with acute lung injury. *Crit Care Med.* 2014;42(6):1480–1486.
78. Briegel J, Forst H, Haller M, et al. Stress doses of hydrocortisone reverse hyperdynamic septic shock: a prospective, randomized, double-blind, single-center study. *Crit Care Med.* 1999;27(4):723–732.
79. Schelling G, Kilger E, Roozendaal B, et al. Stress doses of hydrocortisone, traumatic memories, and symptoms of posttraumatic stress disorder in patients after cardiac surgery: a randomized study. *Biol Psychiatry.* 2004;55(6):627–633.

80. Weis F, Kilger E, Roozendaal B, et al. Stress doses of hydrocortisone reduce chronic stress symptoms and improve health-related quality of life in high-risk patients after cardiac surgery: a randomized study. *J Thorac Cardiovasc Surg.* 2006;131(2):277–282.

81. Boer KR, van Ruler O, van Emmerik AA, et al. Factors associated with posttraumatic stress symptoms in a prospective cohort of patients after abdominal sepsis: a nomogram. *Intensive Care Med.* 2008;34(4):664–674.

82. Schelling G, Roozendaal B, Krauseneck T, et al. Efficacy of hydrocortisone in preventing posttraumatic stress disorder following critical illness and major surgery. *Ann N Y Acad Sci.* 2006;1071:46–53.

83. Pitman RK. Post-traumatic stress disorder, hormones, and memory. *Biol Psychiatry.* 1989;26(3):221–223.

84. McGaugh JL. *Memory and Emotion: The Making of Lasting Memories.* New York: Columbia University Press; 2003.

85. Pitman RK, Delahanty DL. Conceptually driven pharmacologic approaches to acute trauma. *CNS Spectr.* 2005;10(2):99–106.

86. Ekström-Jodal B, Häggendal J, Larsson LE, et al. Cerebral hemodynamics, oxygen uptake and cerebral arteriovenous differences of catecholamines following *E. coli* endotoxin in dogs. *Acta Anaesthesiol Scand.* 1982;26(5):446–452.

87. Ekström-Jodal B, Larsson LE. Effects of dopamine of cerebral circulation and oxygen metabolism in endotoxic shock: an experimental study in dogs. *Crit Care Med.* 1982;10(6):375–377.

88. Sharshar T, Hopkinson NS, Orlikowski D, et al. Science review: the brain in sepsis—culprit and victim. *Crit Care.* 2005;9(1):37–44.

89. Ebersoldt M, Sharshar T, Annane D. Sepsis-associated delirium. *Intensive Care Med.* 2007;33(6):941–950.

90. Siami S, Annane D, Sharshar T. The encephalopathy in sepsis. *Crit Care Clin.* 2008;24(1):67–82.

91. Schelling G. Post-traumatic stress disorder in somatic disease: lessons from critically ill patients. *Prog Brain Res.* 2008;167:229–237.

92. Hauer D, Weis F, Krauseneck T, et al. Traumatic memories, post-traumatic stress disorder and serum cortisol levels in long-term survivors of the acute respiratory distress syndrome. *Brain Res.* 2009;1293:114–120.

93. Furtado M, Katzman MA. Neuroinflammatory pathways in anxiety, posttraumatic stress, and obsessive compulsive disorders. *Psychiatry Res.* 2015;229(1-2):37–48.

94. Weisaeth L. Torture of a Norwegian ship's crew: stress reactions, coping and psychiatric after-effects. In: Wilson JP, Raphael B, eds. *International Handbook of Traumatic Stress Syndromes.* New York: Plenum Press; 1993:743–750.

95. Weisaeth L. A study of behavioural responses to an industrial disaster. *Acta Psychiatr Scand Suppl.* 1989;355:13–24.

96. Weisaeth L. Torture of a Norwegian ship's crew. The torture, stress reactions and psychiatric after-effects. *Acta Psychiatr Scand Suppl.* 1989;355:63–72.

97. First MB, Spitzer RL, Gibbon M, et al. *Structured Clinical Interview for DSM-IV Axis I Disorders.* Washington, DC: American Psychiatric Press; 1996.

98. Schelling G, Kapfhammer HP. Surviving the ICU does not mean that the war is over. *Chest.* 2013;144(1):1–3.

99. Bienvenu OJ, Williams JB, Yang A, et al. Posttraumatic stress disorder in survivors of acute lung injury: evaluating the Impact of Event Scale–Revised. *Chest.* 2013;144(1):24–31.

100. Foa EB. *Posttraumatic Stress Diagnostic Scale Manual.* Eden Prairie, MN: National Computer Systems Inc.; 1995.

101. Weiss DS, Marmar CR. The Impact of Event Scale–Revised. In: Wilson JP, Keane TM, eds. *Assessing Psychological Trauma and PTSD: A Practioner's Handbook.* New York: Guilford Press; 1997:399–411.

102. Blake DD, Weathers FW, Nagy LM, et al. The development of a clinician-administered PTSD scale. *J Trauma Stress.* 1995;8(1):75–90.

103. American Psychiatric Association. *Diagnostic and Statistical Manual of Mental Disorders,* 5th ed. (DSM-5). Washington, DC: American Psychiatric Association; 2013.

104. Gnanavel S, Robert RS. *Diagnostic and Statistical Manual of Mental Disorders,* Fifth Edition, and the Impact of Events Scale–Revised. *Chest.* 2013;144(6):1974.

105. Bienvenu OJ, Needham DM, Hopkins RO. Response. *Chest.* 2013;144(6):1974–1975.

106. Davydow DS, Gifford JM, Desai SV, et al. Depression in general intensive care unit survivors: a systematic review. *Intensive Care Med.* 2009;35(5):796–809.

107. Rabiee A, Nikayin S, Hashem MD, et al. Depressive symptoms after critical illness: a systematic review and meta-analysis. *Crit Care Med.* 2016;44(9):1744–1753.

108. Bienvenu OJ, Colantuoni E, Mendez-Tellez PA, et al. Depressive symptoms and impaired physical function after acute lung injury: a 2-year longitudinal study. *Am J Respir Crit Care Med.* 2012;185(5):517–524.

109. Hopkins RO, Key CW, Suchyta MR, et al. Risk factors for depression and anxiety in survivors of acute respiratory distress syndrome. *Gen Hosp Psychiatry.* 2010;32(2):147–155.

110. Jackson JC, Hart RP, Gordon SM, et al. Six-month neuropsychological outcome of medical intensive care unit patients. *Crit Care Med.* 2003;31(4):1226–1234.

111. Boyle M, Murgo M, Adamson H, et al. The effect of chronic pain on health related quality of life amongst intensive care survivors. *Aust Crit Care.* 2004;17(3):104–113.

112. Guentner K, Hoffman LA, Happ MB, et al. Preferences for mechanical ventilation among survivors of prolonged mechanical ventilation and tracheostomy. *Am J Crit Care.* 2006;15(1):65–77.

113. Weinert C, Meller W. Epidemiology of depression and antidepressant therapy after acute respiratory failure. *Psychosomatics.* 2006;47(5):399–407.

114. Young E, Eddleston J, Ingleby S, et al. Returning home after intensive care: a comparison of symptoms of anxiety and depression in ICU and elective cardiac surgery patients and their relatives. *Intensive Care Med.* 2005;31(1):86–91.

115. Eddleston JM, White P, Guthrie E. Survival, morbidity, and quality of life after discharge from intensive care. *Crit Care Med.* 2000;28(7):2293–2299.

116. Chelluri L, Im KA, Belle SH, et al. Long-term mortality and quality of life after prolonged mechanical ventilation. *Crit Care Med.* 2004;32(1):61–69.

117. Knowles RE, Tarrier N. Evaluation of the effect of prospective patient diaries on emotional well-being in intensive care unit survivors: a randomized controlled trial. *Crit Care Med.* 2009;37(1):184–191.

118. Peek GJ, Mugford M, Tiruvoipati R, et al. Efficacy and economic assessment of conventional ventilatory support versus extracorporeal membrane oxygenation for severe adult respiratory failure (CESAR): a multicentre randomised controlled trial. *Lancet.* 2009;374(9698):1351–1363.

119. Jones C, Eddleston J, McCairn A, et al. Improving rehabilitation after critical illness through outpatient physiotherapy classes and essential amino acid supplement: a randomized controlled trial. *J Crit Care.* 2015;30(5):901–907.

120. Walsh TS, Salisbury LG, Merriweather JL, et al. Increased hospital-based physical rehabilitation and information provision after intensive care unit discharge: the RECOVER randomized clinical trial. *JAMA Intern Med.* 2015;175(6):901–910.

121. Chelluri L, Pinsky MR, Donahoe MP, et al. Long-term outcome of critically ill elderly patients requiring intensive care. *JAMA.* 1993;269(24):3119–3123.

122. Broslawski GE, Elkins M, Algus M. Functional abilities of elderly survivors of intensive care. *J Am Osteopath Assoc.* 1995;95(12):712–717.

123. McWilliams DJ, Atkinson D, Carter A, et al. Feasibility and impact of a structured, exercise-based rehabilitation programme for intensive care survivors. *Physiother Theory Pract.* 2009;25(8):566–571.

124. Rattray J, Crocker C, Jones M, et al. Patients' perceptions of and emotional outcome after intensive care: results from a multicentre study. *Nurs Crit Care.* 2010;15(2):86–93.

125. McKinley S, Aitken LM, Alison JA, et al. Sleep and other factors associated with mental health and psychological distress after intensive care for critical illness. *Intensive Care Med.* 2012;38(4):627–633.

126. Raveau T, Annweiler C, Chudeau N, et al. [Comprehensive geriatric assessment in intensive care unit: a pilot study (pre-Seniorea)]. *Geriatr Psychol Neuropsychiatr Vieil.* 2013;11(4):389–395.

127. Jackson JC, Pandharipande PP, Girard TD, et al. Depression, post-traumatic stress disorder, and functional disability in survivors of critical illness in the BRAIN-ICU study: a longitudinal cohort study. *Lancet Respir Med.* 2014;2(5):369–379.

128. Parsons EC, Hough CL, Vitiello MV, et al. Insomnia is associated with quality of life impairment in medical-surgical intensive care unit survivors. *Heart Lung.* 2015;44(2):89–94.

129. Kowalczyk M, Nestorowicz A, Fijałkowska A, et al. Emotional sequelae among survivors of critical illness: a long-term retrospective study. *Eur J Anaesthesiol.* 2013;30(3):111–118.

130. Battle C, James K, Temblett P. Depression following critical illness: analysis of incidence and risk factors. *J Intensive Care Soc.* 2015;16(2):105–108.

131. Risnes I, Heldal A, Wagner K, et al. Psychiatric outcome after severe cardio-respiratory failure treated with extracorporeal membrane oxygenation: a case-series. *Psychosomatics.* 2013;54(5):418–427.

132. Quality of Life After Mechanized Ventilation in the Elderly Study Investigators. 2-month mortality and functional status of critically ill adult patients receiving prolonged mechanical ventilation. *Chest.* 2002;121(2):549–558.

133. Barr PJ, Thompson R, Walsh T, et al. The psychometric properties of CollaboRATE: a fast and frugal patient-reported measure of the shared decision-making process. *J Med Internet Res.* 2014;16(1):e2.

134. Davydow DS, Russo JE, Ludman E, et al. The association of comorbid depression with intensive care unit admission in patients with diabetes: a prospective cohort study. *Psychosomatics*. 2011;52(2):117–126.

135. Zigmond AS, Snaith RP. The Hospital Anxiety and Depression Scale. *Acta Psychiatr Scand*. 1983;67(6):361–370.

136. Bjelland I, Dahl AA, Haug TT, et al. The validity of the Hospital Anxiety and Depression Scale. An updated literature review. *J Psychosom Res*. 2002;52(2):69–77.

137. Prescott HC, Iwashyna TJ. Somatic symptoms in survivors of critical illness. *Lancet Respir Med*. 2014;2(5):341–343.

138. Jutte JE, Needham DM, Pfoh ER, et al. Psychometric evaluation of the Hospital Anxiety and Depression Scale 3 months after acute lung injury. *J Crit Care*. 2015;30(4):793–798.

139. Stevenson JE, Colantuoni E, Bienvenu OJ, et al. General anxiety symptoms after acute lung injury: predictors and correlates. *J Psychosom Res*. 2013;75(3):287–293.

140. Nikayin S, Rabiee A, Hashem MD, et al. Anxiety symptoms in survivors of critical illness: a systematic review and meta-analysis. *Gen Hosp Psychiatry*. 2016:43:23–29.

141. Davydow DS, Hough CL, Russo JE, et al. The association between intensive care unit admission and subsequent depression in patients with diabetes. *Int J Geriatr Psychiatry*. 2012;27(1):22–30.

142. Davydow DS, Hough CL, Langa KM, et al. Symptoms of depression in survivors of severe sepsis: a prospective cohort study of older Americans. *Am J Geriatr Psychiatry*. 2013;21(9):887–897.

143. Wunsch H, Christiansen CF, Johansen MB, et al. Psychiatric diagnoses and psychoactive medication use among nonsurgical critically ill patients receiving mechanical ventilation. *JAMA*. 2014;311(11):1133–1142.

Rehabilitation Psychology Insights for Treatment of Critical Illness Survivors

JENNIFER E. JUTTE, JAMES C. JACKSON, AND RAMONA O. HOPKINS

INTRODUCTION

As many as one out of every two intensive care unit (ICU) survivors suffers from newly acquired or exacerbated clinically debilitating morbidities that can last years,[1] including physical, cognitive, and psychological disorders that result in functional impairments and reduced quality of life. This cluster of morbidities is known as post–intensive care syndrome (PICS).[2,3] Since the late 1990s, when cognitive deficits and psychological disorders were first recognized in ICU survivors, a primary focus has been on prevention or interventions to improve outcomes. Studies have emphasized the early identification of risk factors in the hope that these risk factors can potentially be modified, contributing to improved long-term outcomes. This is a logical strategy, as key contributors to poor outcomes such as delirium are, to some extent, modifiable. However, some risk factors are demographic in nature (e.g., age or sex) or otherwise cannot be eliminated (e.g., pre-existing illnesses). Since post-ICU cognitive impairment and

psychiatric disorders likely will not be completely preventable, it is important for us to determine how to minimize or treat long-term impairment
and distress. In this chapter, we describe what rehabilitation psychology is
and discuss its relevance to the cognitive and psychiatric problems faced
by survivors of critical illness. Of course, though we emphasize rehabilitation psychology here, we hope that our discussion is useful to all clinicians
who treat critical illness survivors with neuropsychiatric morbidities.

REHABILITATION PSYCHOLOGY

Rehabilitation psychology has been a specialty area of practice for nearly
60 years, with its own board certification since 1997.[4] Traditionally, rehabilitation psychologists have worked with individuals with health conditions that affect neurocognitive, motor, and sensory function across the
continuum of care settings, including intensive care, acute and post-acute
medical rehabilitation settings, private practice, vocational rehabilitation
settings, school settings, and military and veteran's hospitals.[4] The focus
of clinical rehabilitation psychology practice and research is to enhance
health, independence, functional abilities, social role participation, vocational participation, and adjustment among individuals with disabilities
and chronic health conditions.[4]

Relevance of Rehabilitation Psychology to Treatment
of Critical Illness Survivors

Patients who participate in medical rehabilitation often come from an
ICU environment and are recovering from critical illnesses or traumatic
injuries. Critical illnesses and ICU stays can be particularly stressful to
patients, caregivers, and hospital staff. Psychologists who are accus-
tomed to providing services in team-based settings, with a focus on
assisting individuals with newly acquired disabilities and health-related
limitations to adjust to new limitations and reformulate their sense of

personal identity, can be particularly valuable in the ICU setting. During ICU stays patients can experience a wide range of problems, including sleep–wake cycle dysregulation, absence of privacy, communication difficulties that impact their ability to express needs and/or understand and communicate with their providers, lost autonomy, fear and anxiety, depression, confusion and delirium, and pain. Patients admitted to an ICU are particularly vulnerable to psychological distress, both during their ICU stay and hospitalization, as well as long after ICU discharge.[5,6] Because of their training in assessment and intervention practices with individuals suffering from a variety of complex medical conditions, rehabilitation psychologists are particularly well-suited to identify and address the complex post-ICU morbidities faced by ICU survivors across the continuum of care environments (Figure 5.1).

Research over the past 15 years has found—unfortunately—that ICU survivors often do not return to their pre–critical illness baseline level of physical, psychological, or cognitive function. As discussed in previous chapters, the physical, cognitive, and psychiatric symptoms suffered by critical illness survivors are varied and associated with poor quality of life, increased dependency in activities of daily living, transition in family roles, changes in romantic relationships, lifestyle changes, decreased engagement in pleasurable activities, one's ability to return to work, and overall life expectancy.[7-10] Rehabilitation psychologists have the education, training, and experience necessary to work with individuals with impairments in daily function, and they are uniquely qualified to provide care during and after ICU stays that may positively affect engagement in rehabilitation therapies and, therefore, enhance longer-term physical, psychological, and cognitive outcomes. While there are extensive data in other populations such as traumatic brain injury survivors, data are extremely limited on the effects of rehabilitation of cognitive and psychological morbidities in survivors of critical illness. At present, rehabilitation psychologists are too seldom involved in the care of patients in intensive care (in contrast to most trauma care settings). To some extent, this is understandable, since rehabilitation medicine and early physical rehabilitation, such as early mobility, have largely been neglected in ICU environments,

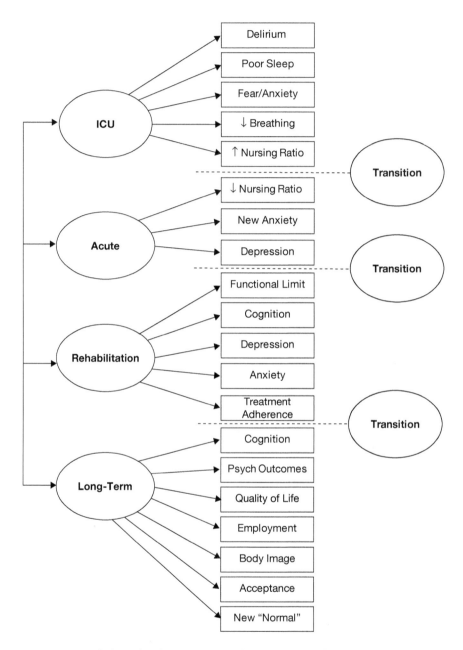

Figure 5.1. Psychological and cognitive considerations across the continuum of care.

particularly in ICUs where the culture still emphasizes that "a patient who is detached from the environment who was woken only on occasions" is an "ideal" patient.[11] As noted in Chapter 2, a more modern view is that critically ill patients should be kept as awake as possible and encouraged to get up, moving, and interacting very early in their ICU course (i.e., engaged in rehabilitation). As a result of a more passive environment, many patients are discharged directly to their homes and communities with few resources, little information, and a high associated cost burden of survivorship.[12] While more ICU patients currently receive early physical rehabilitation and mobilization in the ICU, there has not been a similar rehabilitation emphasis on interventions for cognitive and psychological morbidities after hospital discharge.

COGNITIVE EFFECTS OF CRITICAL ILLNESS

A note about delirium and medical decision-making capacity

In ICUs and acute hospital wards, nonpsychiatric physicians often ask mental health clinicians to assess medical decision-making capacity, although this is something any physician can do.[13] The issue typically comes up when patients demand to leave the hospital against medical advice or refuse recommended treatments. Reduced decision-making capacity can adversely affect a patient's safety and ought to be addressed throughout hospitalization, particularly when the patient has been showing signs of confusion, delirium, or both. Decision-making capacity is important for fostering engagement in the rehabilitation process. It is worth noting that cognitive impairments, including delirium, are common causes of reduced decision-making capacity. The elements of decision-making capacity include (1) the ability to communicate a consistent choice, (2) the ability to understand relevant information communicated by a physician, (3) the ability to appreciate the medical situation and likely consequences of treatment options, and (4) the ability to reason about treatment options.[13] Formal capacity assessment tools are available and can be used for assessing decisional capacity (e.g., MacArthur Competence Assessment Tools for Clinical Research and for Treatment[14]) (Table 5.1).

Cognitive impairment after critical illness—a type of brain injury

Cognitive abilities play a crucial role in daily life, in such wide-ranging tasks as managing money, engaging in effective employment, understanding relational dynamics, overseeing a household, raising children, and many more.[15-18] As such, the impact that cognitive impairment has can be quite profound; when such impairment impacts entire clinical populations, this reflects a public health problem. Such is the case among ICU survivors, nearly half of whom experience a new or exacerbated and, often, clinically debilitating brain injury.[1] Sadly, individuals experiencing these injuries are too often ignored as the insults they experience are unidentified. For a variety of complicated reasons, brain injuries are stereotyped as occurring largely in the context of mechanical events—blows to the head, penetrating injuries—yet there are multiple more subtle pathways through which brains can be injured. As noted in Chapter 3, in critically ill patients, these pathways involve the direct effects of inflammation, hypoxia, delirium, glucose dysregulation, and a host of other mechanisms which invariably lead to cognitive decline, typically of a very abrupt, as opposed to a gradual, nature.

Epidemiology of cognitive impairment after critical illness

As over 30 investigations now show, approximately half of all ICU survivors experience newly acquired or exacerbated, clinically debilitating cognitive impairment secondary to the aforementioned brain injuries[1] (referred to herein as ICU-related long-term cognitive impairment, or ICU-LTCI).[19] This impairment varies both in nature and in duration. For example, after critical illness, individuals demonstrate deficits in attention,

TABLE 5.1   REHABILITATION PSYCHOLOGY ASSESSMENT AND INTERVENTION PRACTICES IN THE ICU

Target Area	Focus of Assessment	Assessment Tools/Strategies	Intervention Practices
Physical function	Fatigue/sleep	Self-report	Environmental/situational modifications; relaxation; distraction; cognitive-behavioral strategies; sleep hygiene; limit nocturnal interruptions; motivational interviewing
	Pain	Clinical interview	
	Mobility engagement	Multidimensional Fatigue Inventory (MFI)	
		Fatigue Severity Scale (FSS)	
		Numeric rating scale for pain	
		Faces scale for pain	
		Behavioral Pain Scale (BPS)	
		Critical-Care Pain Observation Tool (CPOT)	
		Adult Nonverbal Pain Scale (NVPS)	
		Behavioral Pain Scale (BPS)	
		Hopkins Rehabilitation Engagement Rating Scale	
		Rehabilitation Intensity of Therapy Scale (RITS)	
		Pittsburgh Rehab Participation Scale (PRPS)	
Cognitive function	Decisional capacity	CA test of decisional capacity	Capacity assessment (if capacity is limited, determine who the appropriate decision maker is and ensure their decisional capacity); assess for delirium, provide behavioral/environmental recs, consult with primary team and psychiatry; education; brief mental status screening (if impaired, proceed with definitive
	Healthcare literacy	University of California, San Diego, Brief Assessment of Capacity to Consent (UBACC)	
	Delirium	MacArthur Competence Assessment Tools for Clinical Research and for Treatment (MacCAT)	
	Mental status/ neurocognitive function	Healthcare literacy tool	

(continued)

TABLE 5.1 CONTINUED

Target Area	Focus of Assessment	Assessment Tools/Strategies	Intervention Practices
		Confusion Assessment Method–ICU (CAM-ICU)	evaluation); cognitive rehabilitation (compensatory versus restorative)
		Intensive Care Delirium Screening Check List (ICDSC)	
		Mini Mental Status Examination (MMSE) Mini-Cog	
		Montreal Cognitive Assessment (MoCA)	
		Repeatable Battery for the Assessment of Neuropsychological Status (RBANS)	
		Other comprehensive neuropsychological test batteries	
Psychological function	Adjustment	Self-report; clinical interview	CBT-based interventions; calm breathing; guided imagery; engagement in pleasurable activity; environmental modification; mindfulness; symptom management; ICU diaries (PTSD prevention); post-ICU cognitive processing therapy, exposure therapy, EMDR, psychoeducation, cognitive rehabilitation; problem-solving therapy; engagement in early mobility; information regarding positive changes that will occur in physical body or scarring over time
	Anxiety and acute stress	Visual analog anxiety scale	
	Posttraumatic stress disorder (PTSD)	Faces scale	
		State Anxiety Inventory (SAI)	
		Beck Anxiety Inventory (BAI)	
		Hospital Depression and Anxiety Scale (HADS)	
		Psychopathy Check List–Revised (PCL-R)	
	Depression	Impact of Events Scale–Revised (IES-R)	
		Posttraumatic Stress Scale-10 (PTSS-10)	
		Patient Health Questionnaire-9 (PHQ-9)	
		Beck Depression Inventory (BDI) or HADS	
	Body image dissatisfaction	Center for Epidemiologic Studies-Depression (CES-D)	
		Assessment of body image	

Substance use/ abuse	Drug and alcohol use before and after ICU stay Opioid abuse Maladaptive consequences of behaviors	NIDA Drug Use Screening Tool Brief Michigan Alcohol Screening Test (BMAST) Alcohol Use Disorders Identification Test (AUDIT) The CAGE test for alcohol addiction Drug Abuse Screening Test (DAST-10) Alcohol, Smoking and Substance Involvement Screening Test (ASSIST) Inventory of Drug Use Consequences (InDUC-2L)	Motivational interviewing; refer to substance abuse specialists and/or support groups such as AA and NA
Quality of life	Health-related quality of life Disability	Medical Outcomes Study Short Form (SF-36) EuroQol-5D (EQ-5D) World Health Organization Disability Assessment Scale (WHODAS) Sickness Impact Profile (SIP)	Normalization of difficulties; reassurance; instill sense of realistic hope for recovery of function; refer to physical function, cognitive function-ing and psychological function intervention practices

language, memory, processing speed, visual-spatial functioning, and executive ability.[19] Evidence to date suggests that deficits in attention, memory, and executive ability are particularly common, but whether this reflects an actual clinical phenomenon or simply the fact that these abilities have been the most widely studied is unclear.[19] While the natural history of ICU-LTCI is understudied and remains unknown, this condition is widely recognized to be quite long-lasting, and at least one study has documented major decrements in ICU survivors up to 7 years after discharge, suggesting this phenomenon is often permanent.[19]

While cognitive impairment is often associated with advanced age, ICU-LTCI is decidedly not an older-age phenomenon. The BRAIN-ICU study—the largest study conducted to date with over 800 patients—demonstrated that after adjusting for relevant variables, young and older patients performed similarly (that is, poorly) on a cognitive testing battery.[1] While older age may render individuals vulnerable to decline, post-ICU cognitive impairment has been reported in children and is observed in both younger and middle-aged adults. This is a clinically relevant observation, as healthcare providers need to recognize that the nongeriatric patients they work with are, themselves, virtually as susceptible to cognitive changes as their elderly patients might be—decline which, as we outline later in this chapter, may be remediable.

COGNITIVE REHABILITATION IN CRITICAL ILLNESS SURVIVORS

Relatively few survivors of critical illness routinely receive cognitive rehabilitation after ICU discharge. A study in ICU survivors found that only 12% of patients received cognitive rehabilitation after their critical illness. Unfortunately, the majority of rehabilitation is focused on physical morbidities rather than on cognitive impairments.[20] Cognitive rehabilitation is a "systematic, functionally oriented service of therapeutic activities that is based on assessment and understanding of patient's brain-behavioral deficits."[21] Cognitive rehabilitation seeks to achieve functional improvements by (1) reinforcing or re-establishing previously learned behavior patterns or (2) establishing new cognitive activity patterns or compensatory mechanisms for impaired neurological systems.[22] Modern cognitive rehabilitation likely began during World War I, in an effort to treat soldiers surviving increasingly severe head injuries.[23] Current concepts in cognitive rehabilitation emerged during World War II and led to the creation of specialized brain rehabilitation centers. Cognitive rehabilitation is an active field of research, primarily surrounding its use for over 2 million individuals suffering traumatic brain injury (TBI) each year.

A large and growing body of data support using cognitive rehabilitation in the treatment of acquired brain injuries (any noncongenital brain injury—e.g., TBI and stroke).[21,24,25] Three recent systematic reviews of the cognitive rehabilitation literature (nearly 400 studies with 65 graded Class I evidence) found that cognitive rehabilitation was frequently effective in remediating impairments in attention, memory, language and communication, and executive functioning in patients with TBI or stroke.[21,24,25] These studies included therapist-based, group-based, and computer-based interventions, and the data supporting their efficacy with traditionally defined brain-injured populations likely apply to patients with cognitive deficits due to critical illness as well. Indeed, this logic has been the impetus for the use of cognitive rehabilitation with other brain-injured medical populations.

Cognitive rehabilitation in medical populations

Cognitive rehabilitation is increasingly being applied to patients with medical conditions resulting in acquired brain injuries, such as HIV/AIDS, epilepsy, Parkinson's disease, multiple sclerosis, and cancer or "chemo fog."[26-31] A recent review included 34 studies of cognitive rehabilitation in 11 medical illnesses (including anoxia, encephalitis, epilepsy, systemic lupus erythematosus, and brain cancer).[27] The majority of the studies cited in this review were case series or uncontrolled studies, yet 30 of 34 studies demonstrated positive findings. These findings are relevant and

promising for ICU survivors, as they suggest that individuals with significant cognitive disruptions related to medical conditions have the potential
to improve, with some exceptions such as anoxia. While a detailed discussion of cognitive rehabilitation is beyond the scope of this chapter, one
potential example of the use of such an approach with survivors of critical
illness may be instructive here.

Goal management training: enhancing cognitive function following critical illness

Evidence supporting cognitive rehabilitation for executive dysfunction, a
common condition following critical illness, primarily endorses the use of
so-called metacognitive (e.g., thinking about one's thinking) approaches.
These approaches emphasize the development of self-awareness, self-
monitoring, and self-control.[24] The most widely investigated approach
is goal management training (GMT). Based on the theory of "goal
neglect,"[32-34] GMT is a stepwise intervention that uses self-awareness and
self-monitoring techniques to train patients to "stop" and monitor ongoing behavior and regain cognitive control when behavior becomes incom-
patible with intended goals.[35]

Two studies have assessed the efficacy of GMT for cognitive rehabilitation in critical illness survivors, both in the context of physical rehabilitation.[36,37] In the first of these, Jackson and colleagues tested the efficacy of
12 weeks of combined GMT and physical therapy versus usual care in a
randomized pilot feasibility study involving 21 ICU survivors with either
cognitive or functional impairment at hospital discharge. Thirteen participants received the intervention, which involved a combination of tele-
medicine and in-home cognitive, physical, and functional rehabilitation
after hospital discharge. At 3-month follow-up, the intervention group had
significantly better executive functioning compared to the control group,
as assessed with a measure of strategic thinking and planning (the Tower
Test).[36] In addition, the intervention group reported significantly better
functional status. In the second study, a total of 87 critically ill patients

were randomized to usual care, early once-daily physical therapy, or early once-daily physical therapy plus cognitive stimulation which focused on memory, attention, and problem-solving; all interventions were delivered during the acute hospitalization, although a subset of patients also received outpatient GMT after hospital discharge.[37] At 3-month follow-up, there were no differences in cognitive impairment, functional impairment, or health-related quality of life across groups. While we still have much to learn, cognitive rehabilitation—whether GMT or other approaches—merits further consideration in the management of brain-injured survivors of critical illness.

PSYCHOLOGICAL EFFECTS OF CRITICAL ILLNESS

As noted in Chapter 4, critical illnesses and ICU stays often precipitate the development of new psychiatric symptoms or may aggravate pre-existing psychiatric disorders.[38] In addition, psychiatric disorders may increase vulnerability to medical problems, including critical illnesses. For example, a Danish population data-based study of over 24,000 critically ill patients found that a pre-ICU psychiatric diagnosis was associated with an increased risk of developing critical illness.[39]

Psychological factors frequently have a greater impact on rehabilitation and recovery than the medical conditions themselves. Findings from health psychology suggest that individuals with a medical illness perceive their illnesses in the context of five components: (1) the identity or the label the person uses to describe the illness; (2) thoughts and personal explanations about the possible causes of the illness; (3) expectations about the timeline or duration of symptoms; (4) the expected consequences or outcome of the illness; and (5) ways in which the individual believes he or she has power or control over the illness trajectory.[40] This framework can usefully be adopted to describe the trajectory of recovery from critical illness in a rehabilitation environment, positively or adversely impacting one's sense of self; motivation to engage in prescribed treatments; and sense of empowerment and hopefulness.

Psychological distress experienced during an ICU stay can have an adverse impact on post-ICU psychological function[7,41–44] and may also affect physical function due to patients' limited ability to engage in rehabilitation efforts while in the ICU and/or afterward. Pain is another common complaint experienced by individuals who are hospitalized for critical illnesses. Pain can include physiological trauma, such as endotracheal intubation, suctioning, and other intensive care procedures. Critically ill patients often are unable to accurately communicate their pain to clinicians, and they experience sleep–wake cycle dysregulation that can exacerbate their pain experience.

Although we do not yet know the ideal timing of interventions, we believe that prevention and early treatment likely can positively affect not only long-term psychological outcomes but also physical outcomes, through enhanced engagement in early mobilization, which can better prepare patients for active participation in rehabilitation (Table 5.1). Participation in physical activity (e.g., early mobilization) may be associated with reductions in anxiety and depressive symptoms, as physical activity has been shown to be effective in other treatment settings.[45,46] Physical activity increases neurogenesis, with associated improvements in important areas of cognitive function, including learning and memory, both of which are key targets of cognitive rehabilitation.[47] Engagement in early mobility also is likely to positively affect other outcomes such as successful employment, enhanced health-related quality of life, and reduced resource utilization.

Anxiety

General anxiety after critical illness is common, and a number of studies have assessed the incidence of anxiety states. For example, Hopkins and colleagues found that post-ICU anxiety occurred in 23% of survivors.[48] In a review of psychiatric disorders in survivors of acute respiratory distress syndrome (ARDS), the median point prevalence of nonspecific anxiety was 20%.[6] Two recent partially overlapping multicenter studies reported that 42% and 46% of survivors had anxiety at 6-month follow-up, with little improvement at 12 months (42% and 41%, respectively).[20,49] A separate multicenter study found that 38–44% of survivors of acute lung injury reported anxiety, and the symptoms of anxiety were stable over the 24-month follow-up period, with 56% of survivors having anxiety at some point during the 3-, 6-, 12- or 24-month follow-up.[50] Of note, 32% had a remission of anxiety symptoms over the follow-up period, with better physical function associated with anxiety remission and recent impairments in instrumental activities of daily living associated with increased anxiety.[50] In another study using the same cohort, 38% of survivors of acute lung injury experienced general anxiety symptoms, and anxiety symptoms were associated with functional dependence and worse quality of life.[51]

Only a few studies have been conducted to determine the most effective anxiety assessment tools.[52-54] Preferred assessment tools for use in ICU populations are brief, easy and rapid to administer (as patients may become easily fatigued), and straightforward for patients who may have compromised ability to communicate due to endotracheal intubation or sedation, such as visual analog anxiety scales (Table 5.1).[54,55] Studies that incorporate formal diagnostic methods, such as the Structured Clinical Interview for DSM-5 (SCID-5), are also needed.

Few studies have assessed the most effective treatment and non-pharmacological intervention strategies.[56,57] A variety of treatment strategies are used in other settings; however, there are a limited number of studies that have tested these or determined the appropriate frequency or timing of interventions in critically ill populations (Table 5.1). Among the nonpharmacological interventions that have been tested and shown to be helpful in the ICU are randomized trials of nurse-administered music therapy,[56,58] and a pre-post study of nonspecific psychological interventions in an Italian trauma ICU; the latter interventions included supportive psychotherapy, stress management, and educational interventions.[57] In a study that used telephone-based coping skills training for ICU survivors, the intervention was associated with reduced anxiety.[59]

Acute stress disorder

During an ICU stay, treatment of signs of acute stress (i.e., PTSD symptoms that develop within the first month of exposure to critical illness, intensive care, and delirium-related delusions and hallucinations)
includes early management of symptoms (Table 5.1).[60-63] Early management may consist of normalizing symptoms; offering reassurance that the
symptoms are expected to decrease in frequency and intensity over time;
regulation of sleep–wake cycles to the extent possible in a chaotic hospital
environment; and effective pain management while avoiding overuse of
opioid medications, which can have an adverse effect on sleep.[57,64] There
are limited studies of the incidence of these symptoms during or immediately after an ICU stay, or of feasible measures of assessment or viable and
effective treatment approaches (Table 5.1).

Posttraumatic stress disorder

Critical illness survivors frequently develop posttraumatic stress disorder (PTSD).[60,65] In addition to the physical traumas they face, signs
of PTSD among these survivors tend to be related to their hospital
experiences (e.g., frightening memories colored by misinterpretations,
illusions, delusions and hallucinations; being restrained and having
aversive medical procedures done to them while semi-conscious due to
organ failure, benzodiazepine administration), which for many patients
result in avoidance of future medical interventions, thereby precipitating worse physical and perhaps cognitive and psychological outcomes.
Recent partially overlapping multicenter studies found the prevalence
of PTSD was 25% to 26% at 6 months and 23% to 26% at 12 months[49,66]
after hospitalization for ARDS. Two brief screening measures of PTSD
have been cross-validated against clinician diagnosis for use in critical
illness survivor populations: the Impact of Events Scale–Revised (IES-R)
and the Post-Traumatic Stress Syndrome 10-question inventory (PTSS-
10) (Table 5.1).[67]

Psychological intervention is recommended as a first-line treatment for PTSD symptoms, before initiating pharmaceutical alternatives or additions.[68] While symptom management is recommended for signs of acute stress during hospitalization, ICU diaries have been found to be instrumental in reducing the prevalence of post-ICU PTSD among patients and their family members. They are used routinely in Europe (see Chapter 6) but unfortunately are not yet employed routinely in the United States (Table 5.1).[69,70] Following hospitalization, first-line empirically supported treatment options for PTSD include trauma-focused cognitive behavioral interventions, including eye movement desensitization and reprocessing (EMDR), prolonged exposure, and cognitive processing treatments.[71] Of these treatment approaches, exposure therapy or a combination of exposure with cognitive therapy has the strongest evidence base in the outpatient setting.[72] Prolonged exposure also may be effective for treatment of acute stress during hospitalization and in prevention of PTSD,[61,62] although these approaches have not yet been tested in the hospital or afterward with critical illness survivors. Several medications have been shown to be effective for symptom amelioration, including D-cycloserine (when combined with trauma-focused cognitive behavioral therapy),[73–76] propranolol for secondary prevention (possibly),[77] and prazosin for nightmares and sleep disturbances.[78–82] Selective serotonin reuptake inhibitors (SSRIs) can also be used in addition to psychotherapy, although benzodiazepine medications are not indicated for this purpose.[83]

Depression

Depression is a common morbidity in the setting of critical illness and ICU hospitalization, with median point prevalence estimates as high as 28%.[84] Several recent multicenter studies found the prevalence of depression was 37% at 6 months, with no decrease over time (37% at 12 months).[49,66] The high prevalence of depression was confirmed by a systematic review and meta-analysis including 38 studies (4,113 patients), showing that the prevalence of depression was between 29% and 30% at 3-, 6- and 12-month follow-up.[85] Individuals with major depression are more likely to die earlier from health-related conditions such as cardiovascular disease, diabetes, and chronic obstructive pulmonary disease than persons without depression.[86,87] Depressive symptoms may also enhance the risk profile for critical illness through mechanisms such as engagement in maladaptive health behaviors and noncompliance with recommended preventive or treatment options.

No measures of depression or depressive symptoms have yet been validated for use during or after an ICU stay. However, many instruments have been validated in a variety of medical and other populations, including the Center for Epidemiologic Studies Depression Scale (CES-D) and its revision (CESD-R),[88–92] the Patient Health Questionnaire 2-item and 9-item questionnaires,[93,94] the Beck Depression Inventory-II,[95] and the Hospital Anxiety and Depression Scale (HADS) (Table 5.1).[96] The EuroQol is often utilized, although it consists of a single question to assess anxiety/depressive symptoms and really is a measure of general distress rather than of anxiety or depression.[97,98] Although not validated for use during an ICU stay, the HADS has recently been validated for use with survivors of critical illness, but not against a clinician-administered instrument.[97] It seems likely that these tools, used in other disease-specific cohorts, are appropriate for characterizing depression in the context of critical illness. Whether or not they can do so is an empirical question and one that deserves future study.

In a prospective study in 104 ICU survivors, the prevalence of major depression (by SCID criteria) was 16% at 2-month follow-up, and antidepressant use at 2 months occurred in 49% of patients; of the patients with no prior history of depression, 28% had a new prescription for antidepressant medication.[92] There have been no studies of nonpharmacological depression interventions in the ICU, although there is one randomized controlled trial that evaluated a wide array of psychosocial outcomes, including depression, up to 6 months following critical care.[99] In one study, post-ICU physical rehabilitation reduced depression;[100] in another, combined physical rehabilitation and essential amino acid treatment reduced depression.[101] Problem-solving therapy (PST) has been found to be helpful for reducing depressive symptoms in other medical populations (e.g., cardiovascular, diabetes) (Table 5.1).[102,103] Given the importance of enhancing engagement in adaptive health behaviors and compliance with treatment recommendations, strategies such as motivational interviewing or motivational enhancement therapy also could be useful, especially since they are brief and solution-focused approaches.[104] Regarding pharmacological approaches, there is inconsistent evidence that antidepressant medications are safe or effective in treatment of critically ill patients.[92]

Body image dissatisfaction

While critical illness interventions such as tracheostomy and other surgical interventions are essential for survival, these and physically compromising conditions, such as ICU-acquired neuromuscular weakness and related decline in muscle strength, may have a profound negative impact on vital aspects of one's sense of self, body image, and well-being.[105] A study of ICU survivors found that many patients experience emotional effects related to their altered appearance from tracheostomy, tube and central-line placement scars, and striae due to volume overload, all of which may contribute to poor body image.[106] Body image issues among critical illness survivors may very well be similar to those experienced by survivors of traumatic burn injuries. In a study of 79 survivors of burn injuries, female gender and importance of appearance predicted body image dissatisfaction up to 12 months following injury.[107] Indeed, body image dissatisfaction is strongly correlated with both physical and psychological components of quality of life,[108] which in turn could affect other important areas of life, including employment, interpersonal relationships, and mental health. It is possible that assessment of body image satisfaction after ICU treatment, in conjunction with psychotherapy, may help to alleviate long-term psychological distress (Table 5.1).

FUNCTIONAL IMPACT OF CRITICAL ILLNESS

Survivors of critical illness frequently experience psychological distress, with an associated adverse impact on physical, social, and vocational function as well as quality of life.[6,84,109–111] Although exposure to the ICU environment may be brief for many patients (e.g., in routine observation after a surgical procedure), increasing concern has focused on patients with longer and more complicated critical illnesses (e.g., ARDS or severe sepsis), including those with chronic critical illness (CCI). These individuals often require weeks to months of assisted breathing via mechanical ventilation (MV) after acute illnesses such as sepsis, and individuals requiring prolonged MV develop functional dependencies, which may include assistance with feeding, bathing, grooming, dressing, bowel and bladder care, transfers, or mobility.[112–114] ICU survivors often experience functional declines. An observational cohort study of survivors of severe sepsis found that 65% of survivors reported severe or complete functional dependency (i.e., dependent with activities of daily living [ADL] which involve self-care—e.g., bathing, dressing, grooming, toileting) 12 months after hospitalization.[112] This is concerning not only for the quality of life of the patient but also for the undue burden this may place on family caregivers.

Functional dependency often translates into significant vocational difficulties. For example, functional dependencies can result in a delay in return to employment after critical illness. Almost half of ICU survivors have not returned to work 12 months after they leave the hospital.[10,48,115] Rehabilitation psychologists are often involved in vocational assessment, which can incorporate educational attainment, aptitude, academic achievement, personality, vocational interests, personal values, and financial needs. Adjustment to critical illness–related disability may be necessary and can impact one's ability to return to one's former occupation. The focus of rehabilitation psychology can be on identifying factors that may facilitate or hinder one's ability to return to previous employment and identifying accommodations and compensatory strategies that may help the individual to be successful when he or she returns to work. Workplace accommodation needs will vary by individual and will depend on the type and extent of physical, cognitive, and emotional effects from the medical condition.

In addition to dealing with functional dependencies and vocational hindrances, survivors of critical illness often are faced with the crucial task of modifying and changing health-related behaviors that (a) are ingrained and long-standing and (b) are not easily amenable to change, especially during a stressful situation such as recovery from critical illness. Persons who are hospitalized with critical illnesses may have a history of engaging in behaviors detrimental to health and well-being, such as smoking, substance or alcohol misuse, poor nutrition, nonadherence to recommended prevention and treatment regimens, and other lifestyle factors compromising their physical condition. Rehabilitation psychologists are equipped to assess and treat health-related behaviors that may limit effective engagement in medical rehabilitation and recovery from critical illness.

SOCIAL SUPPORT

Although we suspect that the benefits of social support are innumerable and far-reaching, the types and amount of social support that are ideal for improving outcomes from critical illness have not yet been explored. Based on information gleaned from the extant, non–critical care literature, it is likely that patients who feel less connected interpersonally may be at risk for development or exacerbation of infections, difficulty with health-related treatments, engagement in health-damaging behaviors, and rehospitalization down the road.[116] A recent cross-sectional study from the Netherlands found that emotional and instrumental support in particular were helpful for post-ICU physical function, and discrepancies between expected and received support had a negative effect on emotional well-being and the psychological dimension of quality of life.[117] Although in this study, patients tended to prefer that all types of social support be provided by a family member rather than their healthcare providers, one way in which perceived social support could be enhanced during hospitalization is through enhanced communication and interactions with clinical providers.

REHABILITATION CASE STUDIES

Early intervention may be key for enhancing emotional, cognitive, and physical function and thus may also enhance the rehabilitation and recovery processes among survivors of critical illness. Here we provide two illustrative case studies.

Case example 1: Cognitive rehabilitation

Mr. Y is a 61-year-old Caucasian man and a recent transplant recipient who was treated after a long hospitalization in the medical ICU, where he experienced a complex course of illness of 30 days' duration that included bouts of sepsis and ARDS. He had been a nurse prior to his transplant, a high-functioning individual with 16 years of education who was fully independent and successful in his various roles. Following the critical illness and the associated long hospital stay, he experienced significant problems that he characterized as memory difficulties, although on closer inspection these difficulties were more reflective of deficits in attention. His problems were exemplified by an event that was very concerning to him: he was at the medical center for one of many routine follow-up appointments and was instructed to stop by the hospital pharmacy to pick up a long list of necessary medications before going home. Instead, he walked past the pharmacy and, along with his informal caregiver, got into his car to make the 100-mile drive to his rural community. He had driven about 60 miles when he realized he was missing his medications, prompting him to return to the hospital to retrieve them.

While Mr. Y was adamant that he was having significant memory problems, a neuropsychological assessment of his memory found no significant memory impairments and, indeed, that his deficits were actually related to significant problems with concentration and sustained attention. He was so preoccupied with worries about his health and his future that he was not actively thinking about the tasks at hand. Given the primacy of his attentional problems, he was believed to be a good candidate for goal management training (GMT), a widely used rehabilitation method effective in the treatment of attention and executive functioning. He completed a 12-week GMT protocol and appeared to benefit, in particular, from techniques involving "absent-minded slips" and "stop-think" (core features of GMT).

"Absent-minded slips" are defined in GMT as careless mistakes that individuals make—for example, walking past a pharmacy window without picking up medication—due to attentional failures (although there are many other potential reasons for such slips). In the logic of GMT, these slips are predictable—that is, they typically occur when individuals are tired, stressed, rushing, or otherwise preoccupied. The challenge for Mr. Y, as with similar patients, was to identify the unique circumstances in which he was most vulnerable to making such slips. For him, these circumstances involved being in a hurry and worrying about his health. When these things happened concurrently, he was particularly vulnerable to making mistakes.

Having gained insight into his propensity to "absent-minded slips," Mr. Y then applied "stop-think." "Stop-think" is a two-step process by which individuals stop themselves in the moment and think about the goals they need to achieve at the time. He began regularly implementing "stop-think" at the grocery store, at the hospital, while running errands, and virtually everywhere he went, being particularly careful to use this technique during times of stress. For example, before leaving the local grocery store, he would perform a quick mental inventory to make sure he had picked up the items he needed. Similarly, when working with his daughter on Social Security disability forms, he would stop and review them regularly, making sure that he did not make careless errors or omissions that would delay the disability adjudication process. Over a 3-month rehabilitation period, he learned to consistently integrate the simple, yet crucial, concepts of GMT, resulting in greater confidence and efficiency and fewer mistakes.

Case example 2: Psychological rehabilitation

Mr. X is a 42-year-old single man who was admitted to the medical intensive care unit (MICU) at a large non-profit university-affiliated teaching hospital. This 16-bed MICU is a critical care unit in which patients who are medically stable enough to participate in medical rehabilitation are provided reduced sedation and early rehabilitation (physical therapy, occupational therapy, and/or speech and language pathology) services. Mr. X was admitted to the MICU for respiratory failure associated with atypical pneumonia. He had been previously healthy with no history of chronic medical or mental health concerns or major injuries. He denied a history of substance or alcohol abuse or dependence. Mr. X spent nearly 3 months in the MICU; an average length of stay is about 4 days.

The initial rehabilitation psychology consultation for Mr. X was for concerns pertaining to anxiety and nonadherence to treatment recommendations, as well as regarding his overall adjustment to and coping with his medical condition and hospitalization. The medical team was concerned that anxiety might be adversely affecting active participation in his prescribed therapies and his ability to be successfully weaned off mechanical ventilation. The team also noted that motivational factors may have contributed to his refusal to participate in his prescribed physical therapy. Mr. X had refused sessions with his physical therapists, which, in addition to his difficulty in getting off mechanical ventilation, prompted the referral to rehabilitation psychology. During the initial assessment and several follow-up sessions, he demonstrated poor awareness of the extent of his physical compromise, believing that he could simply be discharged to his home immediately, where he thought he would have access to a ventilator and resume living with his family.

The primary referral question was whether anxiety could be hindering important aspects of this patient's recovery from critical illness—namely, participation in physical therapy and weaning off mechanical ventilation. When working with patients who are critically ill and mechanically ventilated, there are several key factors to consider:

(1) Communication from the patient to clinicians often must be done through alternative nonverbal modes—in this case, Mr. X communicated through the use of a Portex blue line ultra-suction aid with talk attachment (a.k.a., a "talking trach"), mouthing words, writing, using head nods and shakes to indicate "yes" or "no," and making a thumbs up or down.

(2) Given difficulties in communicating, as well as severity of illness, it was important to co-treat with nursing, speech and language pathology, and respiratory therapy.

(3) For some patients, placement of a speaking valve must only be performed by a respiratory therapist or speech language pathologist. Therefore, sessions were scheduled in coordination with these individuals.

(4) If patients are on pressure support modes of ventilation, they have some control over the *rate* of respirations but not their *depth*. Therefore, any breathing retraining exercises must account for this (e.g., for anxiety or stress management purposes).

(5) There is a constant flow of individuals entering the patient's room at any given moment, from nursing staff to respiratory therapists, and thus any assessment or intervention must account for interruptions.

(6) Patients who are critically ill often suffer from bouts of delirium. Therefore, mental status must be assessed at least twice daily (by the critical care medical team and/or psychologist), not only to determine the patient's ability to participate in psychotherapy interventions but also to continuously monitor for any signs of new infection or problematic dosing of potentially deliriogenic medications.

Patients who are critically ill, physically compromised, and in the ICU environment tend to experience physical, cognitive, and emotional fatigue affecting aspects of their care. As such, the assessment and interventions must be brief. The psychologist met with Mr. X for no more than 30 minutes throughout his ICU stay, and many of the "interventions" involved communicating and collaborating with the treatment team. The development of rapport with the patient, while ensuring a collaborative team approach, was essential in the assessment and treatment and eventual positive outcome of this case.

The interventions were based on cognitive-behavioral therapy (CBT), which is a first-line, efficacious treatment approach adapted from the outpatient setting.[118-123] The treatment included the following CBT elements:

(1) Establishment of rapport/therapeutic alliance
(2) Anxiety psychoeducation (including the impact anxiety can have on respiratory and physical function) based on the biopsychosocial model of anxiety; this included provision of accurate information regarding the nature of sympathetic nervous system arousal, or physiological "sensations," in which Mr. X was taught that the panic he described includes sensations which are normal and harmless
(3) Reflective listening and supportive statements
(4) Normalization of his emotional reaction
(5) Fostering of a sense of hope through reassurance
(6) Exposure to anxious thoughts and feelings
(7) Cognitive restructuring
(8) Relaxation training
(9) Directive statements
(10) Problem-solving
(11) Provision of coping strategies
(12) Relaxation training (calm breathing, guided imagery).

Given that Mr. X was on a type of mechanical ventilation that allows a patient to control the *rate* but not *depth* of breaths, he was encouraged to engage in a "calming" breathing strategy, rather than a diaphragmatic or "deep" breathing approach. Using a calm yet directive voice and interaction style, the psychologist asked him to take a few nice, calm breaths and

focus on how good that felt. His anxiety was assessed using a visual ana-
logue anxiety scale (VAS-A) both before and after the treatment. In addition, he was asked to describe what it felt like to breathe independently
(i.e., before mechanical ventilation) and to imagine this feeling during the
breathing training.

Throughout his hospitalization, there were several key areas of
assessment and intervention that were addressed by the rehabilitation
psychologist:

(1) Assessment—adjustment to new medical diagnosis,
     compromised physical function, hospitalization, and
     rehabilitation; extent and nature of disability and preserved
     abilities; emotional adjustment; and social/behavioral
     functioning
(2) Intervention—anxiety management in the context of weaning
     from mechanical ventilation; motivational enhancement
     treatment for engagement in his prescribed therapies;
     behavioral management for adherence to medical treatment,
     nursing care, and participation in his prescribed therapies;
     adjustment to medical diagnosis and disability; and
     psychoeducation on anxiety as well as his medical diagnosis,
     treatment, and prognosis
(3) Consultation with the critical care medicine rehabilitation team
     was provided for behavioral functioning and psychosocial
     concerns.

SUMMARY: THE ROLE OF THE REHABILITATION PSYCHOLOGIST IN THE ICU

Since post-ICU cognitive and psychiatric difficulties will not be preventable altogether, it is important to attempt to prevent or minimize long-
term impairment and distress. Given the thorough training in assessment
of and intervention practices for patients with a variety of complex

medical conditions, rehabilitation psychologists are particularly well-suited to identify and address the complex post-ICU morbidities faced by critical illness survivors across the continuum of care environments. Interventions across settings to minimize delirium, reduce psychological distress, and shore up cognitive deficits have the capacity to positively influence patients' recovery trajectories and quality of life.

REFERENCES

1. Pandharipande PP, Girard TD, Jackson JC, et al. Long-term cognitive impairment after critical illness. *N Engl J Med*. 2013;369(14):1306–1316.
2. Elliott D, Davidson JE, Harvey MA, et al. Exploring the scope of post–intensive care syndrome therapy and care: engagement of non–critical care providers and survivors in a second stakeholders meeting. *Crit Care Med*. 2014;42(12):2518–2526.
3. Needham DM, Davidson J, Cohen H, et al. Improving long-term outcomes after discharge from intensive care unit: report from a stakeholders' conference*. *Crit Care Med*. 2012;40(2):502–509.
4. Frank RG, Elliott TR. *Handbook of Rehabilitation Psychology*. Washington, DC: American Psychological Association; 2000.
5. Jackson J, Pandharipande P, Girard T. Bringing to light the Risk Factors And Incidence of Neuropsychological dysfunction in ICU survivors (BRAIN-ICU) study investigators: depression, post-traumatic stress disorder, and functional disability in survivors of critical illness in the BRAIN-ICU study: a longitudinal cohort study. *Lancet Respir Med*. 2014;2:369–379.
6. Davydow DS, Desai SV, Needham DM, et al. Psychiatric morbidity in survivors of the acute respiratory distress syndrome: a systematic review. *Psychosom Med*. 2008;70(4):512–519.
7. Desai SV, Law TJ, Needham DM. Long-term complications of critical care. *Crit Care Med* 2011;39(2):371–379.
8. Iwashyna TJ, Ely EW, Smith DM, et al. Long-term cognitive impairment and functional disability among survivors of severe sepsis. *JAMA*. 2010;304(16):1787–1794.
9. Barnato AE, Albert SM, Angus DC, et al. Disability among elderly survivors of mechanical ventilation. *Am J Respir Crit Care Med*. 2011;183(8):1037–1042.
10. Herridge MS, Tansey CM, Matté A, et al. Functional disability 5 years after acute respiratory distress syndrome. *N Engl J Med*. 2011;364(14):1293–1304.
11. Merriman H. The techniques used to sedate ventilated patients. *Intensive Care Med*. 1981;7(5):217–224.
12. Iwashyna TJ, Cooke CR, Wunsch H, et al. Population burden of long-term survivorship after severe sepsis in older Americans. *J Am Geriatr Soc*. 2012;60(6):1070–1077.
13. Appelbaum PS. Assessment of patients' competence to consent to treatment. *N Engl J Med*. 2007;357(18):1834–1840.

14. Dunn LB, Nowrangi MA, Palmer BW, et al. Assessing decisional capacity for clinical research or treatment: a review of instruments. *Am J Psychiatry.* 2006;163(8):1323–1334.

15. Boyle PA, Cohen RA, Paul R, et al. Cognitive and motor impairments predict functional declines in patients with vascular dementia. *Int J Geriatr Psychiatry.* 2002;17(2):164–169.

16. Cahn-Weiner DA, Boyle PA, Malloy PF. Tests of executive function predict instrumental activities of daily living in community-dwelling older individuals. *Appl Neuropsychol.* 2002;9(3):187–191.

17. Boyle PA, Paul RH, Moser DJ, et al. Executive impairments predict functional declines in vascular dementia. *Clin Neuropsychol* 2004;18(1):75–82.

18. Boyle PA, Malloy PF, Salloway S, et al. Executive dysfunction and apathy predict functional impairment in Alzheimer disease. *Am J Geriatr Psychiatry.* 2003;11(2):214–221.

19. Wilcox ME, Brummel NE, Archer K, et al. Cognitive dysfunction in ICU patients: risk factors, predictors, and rehabilitation interventions. *Crit Care Med.* 2013;41(9):S81–S98.

20. Needham DM, Dinglas VD, Bienvenu OJ, et al. One year outcomes in patients with acute lung injury randomised to initial trophic or full enteral feeding: prospective follow-up of EDEN randomised trial. *BMJ.* 2013;346:f1532.

21. Cicerone KD, Dahlberg C, Malec JF, et al. Evidence-based cognitive rehabilitation: updated review of the literature from 1998 through 2002. *Arch Phys Med Rehabil.* 2005;86(8):1681–1692.

22. Harley J, Allen C, Braciszewski T, et al. Guidelines for cognitive rehabilitation. *NeuroRehabilitation.* 1992;2(3):62–67.

23. Boake C. History of cognitive rehabilitation following head injury. In: Kreutzer JS, Wehman PH, eds. *Cognitive Rehabilitation for Persons with Traumatic Brain Injury: A Functional Approach.* Baltimore: Paul C. Brookes; 1991:3–12.

24. Cicerone KD, Langenbahn DM, Braden C, et al. Evidence-based cognitive rehabilitation: updated review of the literature from 2003 through 2008. *Arch Phys Med Rehabil.* 2011;92(4):519–530.

25. Cicerone KD, Dahlberg C, Kalmar K, et al. Evidence-based cognitive rehabilitation: recommendations for clinical practice. *Arch Phys Med Rehabil.* 2000;81(12):1596–1615.

26. Schuurs A, Green HJ. A feasibility study of group cognitive rehabilitation for cancer survivors: enhancing cognitive function and quality of life. *Psycho-Oncology.* 2013;22(5):1043–1049.

27. Langenbahn DM, Ashman T, Cantor J, et al. An evidence-based review of cognitive rehabilitation in medical conditions affecting cognitive function. *Arch Phys Med Rehabil.* 2013;94(2):271–286.

28. Cherrier M, Anderson K, David D, et al. A randomized trial of cognitive rehabilitation in cancer survivors. *Life Sci.* 2013;93(17):617–622.

29. Weber E, Blackstone K, Woods SP. Cognitive neurorehabilitation of HIV-associated neurocognitive disorders: a qualitative review and call to action. *Neuropsychol Rev.* 2013;23(1):81–98.

30. O'Brien SM, Scott LV, Dinan TG. Cytokines: abnormalities in major depression and implications for pharmacological treatment. *Hum Psychopharmacol.* 2004; 19(6):397–403.

31. Pu S, Nakagome K, Yamada T, et al. A pilot study on the effects of cognitive remediation on hemodynamic responses in the prefrontal cortices of patients with schizophrenia: a multi-channel near-infrared spectroscopy study. *Schizophr Res.* 2014;153(1):87–95.

32. Duncan J, Emslie H, Williams P, et al. Intelligence and the frontal lobe: the organization of goal-directed behavior. *Cogn Psychol.* 1996;30(3):257–303.

33. Duncan J, Parr A, Woolgar A, et al. Goal neglect and Spearman's g: competing parts of a complex task. *J Exp Psychol Gen.* 2008;137(1):131.

34. Nieuwenhuis S, Broerse A, Nielen MM, et al. A goal activation approach to the study of executive function: an application to antisaccade tasks. *Brain Cogn.* 2004;56(2):198–214.

35. Levine B, Schweizer TA, O'Connor C, et al. Rehabilitation of executive functioning in patients with frontal lobe brain damage with goal management training. *Front Hum Neurosci.* 2011;5:9.

36. Jackson J, Ely EW, Morey MC, et al. Cognitive and physical rehabilitation of ICU survivors: results of the RETURN randomized, controlled pilot investigation. *Crit Care Med.* 2012;40(4):1088.

37. Brummel N, Girard T, Ely E, et al. Feasibility and safety of early combined cognitive and physical therapy for critically ill medical and surgical patients: the Activity and Cognitive Therapy in ICU (ACT-ICU) trial. *Intensive Care Med.* 2014;40(3):370–379.

38. Bergbom-Engberg I, Haljamae H. Assessment of patients' experience of discomforts during respirator therapy. *Crit Care Med.* 1989;17(10):1068–1072.

39. Wunsch H, Christiansen CF, Johansen MB, et al. Psychiatric diagnoses and psychoactive medication use among nonsurgical critically ill patients receiving mechanical ventilation. *JAMA.* 2014;311(11):1133–1142.

40. Petrie KJ, Weinman J, Sharpe N, et al. Role of patients' view of their illness in predicting return to work and functioning after myocardial infarction: longitudinal study. *BMJ.* 1996;312(7040):1191–1194.

41. Schelling G, Stoll C, Haller M, et al. Health-related quality of life and posttraumatic stress disorder in survivors of the acute respiratory distress syndrome. *Crit Care Med.* 1998;26(4):651–659.

42. Jones C, Griffiths RD, Humphris G, et al. Memory, delusions, and the development of acute posttraumatic stress disorder-related symptoms after intensive care. *Crit Care Med.* 2001;29(3):573–580.

43. Kamdar BB, Needham DM, Collop NA. Sleep deprivation in critical illness: its role in physical and psychological recovery. *J Intensive Care Med.* 2012;27(2):97–111.

44. Davydow DS, Zatzick DF, Rivara FP, et al. Predictors of posttraumatic stress disorder and return to usual major activity in traumatically injured intensive care unit survivors. *Gen Hosp Psychiatry.* 2009;31(5):428–435.

45. Emery CF, Leatherman NE, Burker E, et al. Psychological outcomes of a pulmonary rehabilitation program. *Chest.* 1991;100(3):613–617.

46. Emery CF, Schein RL, Hauck ER, et al. Psychological and cognitive outcomes of a randomized trial of exercise among patients with chronic obstructive pulmonary disease. *Health Psychol.* 1998;17(3):232.

47. Hopkins RO, Suchyta MR, Farrer TJ, et al. Improving post–intensive care unit neuropsychiatric outcomes: understanding cognitive effects of physical activity. *Am J Respir Crit Care Med.* 2012;186(12):1220–1228.

48. Hopkins RO, Weaver LK, Collingridge D, et al. Two-year cognitive, emotional, and quality-of-life outcomes in acute respiratory distress syndrome. *Am J Respir Crit Care Med.* 2005;171(4):340–347.

49. Dinglas VD, Hopkins RO, Wozniak AW, et al. One-year outcomes of rosuvastatin versus placebo in sepsis-associated acute respiratory distress syndrome: prospective follow-up of SAILS randomised trial. *Thorax.* 2016:71(5):401–410.

50. Bienvenu OJ, Colantuoni E, Mendez-Tellez PA, et al. Cooccurrence of and remission from general anxiety, depression, and posttraumatic stress disorder symptoms after acute lung injury: a 2-year longitudinal study. *Crit Care Med.* 2015;43(3):642–653.

51. Stevenson JE, Colantuoni E, Bienvenu OJ, et al. General anxiety symptoms after acute lung injury: predictors and correlates. *J Psychosom Res.* 2013;75(3):287–293.

52. Benotsch EG, Lutgendorf SK, Watson D, et al. Rapid anxiety assessment in medical patients: evidence for the validity of verbal anxiety ratings. *Ann Behavioral Med* 2000;22(3):199–203.

53. Chlan LL. Relationship between two anxiety instruments in patients receiving mechanical ventilatory support. *J Adv Nurs.* 2004;48(5):493–499.

54. McKinley S, Madronio C. Validity of the Faces Anxiety Scale for the assessment of state anxiety in intensive care patients not receiving mechanical ventilation. *J Psychosom Res.* 2008;64(5):503–507.

55. Chlan L, Savik K, Weinert C. Development of a shortened state anxiety scale from the Spielberger State-Trait Anxiety Inventory (STAI) for patients receiving mechanical ventilatory support. *J Nurs Meas.* 2003;11(3):283–293.

56. Chlan LL, Weinert CR, Heiderscheit A, et al. Effects of patient-directed music intervention on anxiety and sedative exposure in critically ill patients receiving mechanical ventilatory support: a randomized clinical trial. *JAMA.* 2013;309(22):2335–2344.

57. Peris A, Bonizzoli M, Iozzelli D, et al. Early intra-intensive care unit psychological intervention promotes recovery from post traumatic stress disorders, anxiety and depression symptoms in critically ill patients. *Crit Care.* 2011;15(1):R41.

58. Wong HL, Lopez-Nahas V, Molassiotis A. Effects of music therapy on anxiety in ventilator-dependent patients. *Heart Lung.* 2001;30(5):376–387.

59. Cox CE, Porter LS, Hough CL, et al. Development and preliminary evaluation of a telephone-based coping skills training intervention for survivors of acute lung injury and their informal caregivers. *Intensive Care Med.* 2012;38(8):1289–1297.

60. Parker AM, Sricharoenchai T, Raparla S, et al. Posttraumatic stress disorder in critical illness survivors: a meta-analysis. *Crit Care Med.* 2015;43(5):1121–1129.

61. Cukor J, Spitalnick J, Difede J, et al. Emerging treatments for PTSD. *Clin Psychol Rev.* 2009;29(8):715–726.

62. Kearns MC, Ressler KJ, Zatzick D, et al. Early interventions for PTSD: a review. *Depress Anxiety*. 2012;29(10):833–842.
63. Garrouste-Orgeas M, Coquet I, Perier A, et al. Impact of an intensive care unit diary on psychological distress in patients and relatives*. *Crit Care Med*. 2012;40(7):2033–2040.
64. Dimsdale JE, Norman D, DeJardin D, et al. The effect of opioids on sleep architecture. *J Clin Sleep Med*. 2007;3(1):33–36.
65. Davydow DS, Gifford JM, Desai SV, et al. Posttraumatic stress disorder in general intensive care unit survivors: a systematic review. *Gen Hosp Psychiatry*. 2008;30(5):421–434.
66. Needham DM, Dinglas VD, Morris PE, et al. Physical and cognitive performance of patients with acute lung injury 1 year after initial trophic versus full enteral feeding. EDEN trial follow-up. *Am J Respir Crit Care Med* 2013;188(5):567–576.
67. Bienvenu OJ, Williams JB, Yang A, et al. Posttraumatic stress disorder in survivors of acute lung injury: evaluating the Impact of Event Scale–Revised. *Chest*. 2013;144(1):24–31.
68. National Collaborating Centre for Mental Health (UK). Post-Traumatic Stress Disorder: The Management of PTSD in Adults and Children in Primary and Secondary Care. Leicester: Gaskell; 2005.
69. Jones C, Bäckman C, Griffiths RD. Intensive care diaries and relatives' symptoms of posttraumatic stress disorder after critical illness: a pilot study. *Am J Crit Care*. 2012;21(3):172–176.
70. Jones C, Backman C, Capuzzo M, et al. Intensive care diaries reduce new-onset post-traumatic stress disorder following critical illness: a randomised, controlled trial. *Crit Care*. 2010;14(5):R168.
71. Forbes D, Creamer M, Bisson JI, et al. A guide to guidelines for the treatment of PTSD and related conditions. *J Trauma Stress*. 2010;23(5):537–552.
72. Powers MB, Halpern JM, Ferenschak MP, et al. A meta-analytic review of prolonged exposure for posttraumatic stress disorder. *Clin Psychol Rev*. 2010;30(6):635–641.
73. Davis M, Ressler K, Rothbaum BO, et al. Effects of D-cycloserine on extinction: translation from preclinical to clinical work. *Biol Psychiatry*. 2006;60(4):369–375.
74. Davis M, Barad M, Otto M, et al. Combining pharmacotherapy with cognitive behavioral therapy: traditional and new approaches. *J Trauma Stress*. 2006; 19(5):571–581.
75. Ledgerwood L, Richardson R, Cranney J. D-cycloserine facilitates extinction of learned fear: effects on reacquisition and generalized extinction. *Biol Psychiatry*. 2005;57(8):841–847.
76. Walker DL, Ressler KJ, Lu KT, et al. Facilitation of conditioned fear extinction by systemic administration or intra-amygdala infusions of D-cycloserine as assessed with fear-potentiated startle in rats. *J Neurosci*. 2002;22(6):2343–2351.
77. Pitman RK, Sanders KM, Zusman RM, et al. Pilot study of secondary prevention of posttraumatic stress disorder with propranolol. *Biol Psychiatry*. 2002;51(2):189–192.
78. Taylor HR, Freeman MK, Cates ME. Prazosin for treatment of nightmares related to posttraumatic stress disorder. *Am J Health Syst Pharm*. 2008;65(8):716–722.

79. Miller LJ. Prazosin for the treatment of posttraumatic stress disorder sleep disturbances. *Pharmacotherapy*. 2008;28(5):656–666.
80. Taylor FB, Martin P, Thompson C, et al. Prazosin effects on objective sleep measures and clinical symptoms in civilian trauma posttraumatic stress disorder: a placebo-controlled study. *Biol Psychiatry*. 2008;63(6):629–632.
81. Raskind MA, Peskind ER, Hoff DJ, et al. A parallel group placebo controlled study of prazosin for trauma nightmares and sleep disturbance in combat veterans with post-traumatic stress disorder. *Biol Psychiatry*. 2007;61(8):928–934.
82. Raskind MA, Peskind ER, Kanter ED, et al. Reduction of nightmares and other PTSD symptoms in combat veterans by prazosin: a placebo-controlled study. *Am J Psychiatry*. 2003;160(2):371–373.
83. Bernardy NC, Friedman MJ. Psychopharmacological strategies in the management of posttraumatic stress disorder (PTSD): what have we learned? *Curr Psychiatry Rep*. 2015;17(4):564.
84. Davydow DS, Gifford JM, Desai SV, et al. Depression in general intensive care unit survivors: a systematic review. *Intensive Care Med*. 2009;35(5):796–809.
85. Rabiee A, Nikayin S, Hashem MD, et al. Depressive symptoms after critical illness: a systematic review and meta-analysis. *Crit Care Med*. 2016;44(9):1744–1753.
86. Chang CK, Hayes RD, Broadbent M, et al. All-cause mortality among people with serious mental illness (SMI), substance use disorders, and depressive disorders in southeast London: a cohort study. *BMC Psychiatry*. 2010;10:77.
87. Katon WJ. Epidemiology and treatment of depression in patients with chronic medical illness. *Dialogues Clinical Neurosci*. 2011;13(1):7–23.
88. Radloff LS. The CES-D scale: a self-report depression scale for research in the general population. *Appl Psychol Meas*. 1977;1(3):385–401.
89. Devins GM, Orme CM, Costello CG, et al. Measuring depressive symptoms in illness populations: psychometric properties of the Center for Epidemiologic Studies Depression (CES-D) scale. *Psychol Health*. 1988;2(2):139–156.
90. Eaton W, Muntaner C, Smith C, et al. Revision of the Center for Epidemiologic Studies Depression (CES-D) Scale. Baltimore, MD: Johns Hopkins University Prevention Center; 1998.
91. Eaton WW, Smith C, Ybarra M, et al. Center for Epidemiologic Studies Depression Scale: review and revision (CESD and CESD-R). Baltimore, MD: Johns Hopkins University Prevention Center; 2004.
92. Weinert C, Meller W. Epidemiology of depression and antidepressant therapy after acute respiratory failure. *Psychosomatics*. 2006;47(5):399–407.
93. Kroenke K, Spitzer RL, Williams JB. The PHQ-9: validity of a brief depression severity measure. *J Gen Internal Med*. 2001;16(9):606–613.
94. Kroenke K, Spitzer RL, Williams JB. The Patient Health Questionnaire-2: validity of a two-item depression screener. *Med Care*. 2003;41(11):1284–1292.
95. Viljoen JL, Iverson GL, Griffiths S, et al. Factor structure of the Beck Depression Inventory-II in a medical outpatient sample. *J Clin Psychol Med Settings*. 2003;10(4):289–291.
96. Zigmond AS, Snaith RP. The Hospital Anxiety and Depression Scale. *Acta Psychiatr Scand*. 1983;67(6):361–370.

97. Jutte JE, Needham DM, Pfoh ER, et al. Psychometric evaluation of the Hospital Anxiety and Depression Scale 3 months after acute lung injury. *J Crit Care.* 2015;30(4):793–798.

98. EuroQol Group. EuroQol—a new facility for the measurement of health-related quality of life. Health Policy. 1990;16(3):199–208.

99. Jones C, Skirrow P, Griffiths RD, et al. Rehabilitation after critical illness: a randomized, controlled trial. *Crit Care Med.* 2003;31(10):2456–2461.

100. McWilliams D, Atkinson D, Carter A, et al. Feasibility and impact of a structured, exercise-based rehabilitation programme for intensive care survivors. *Physiother Theory Pract.* 2009;25(8):566–571.

101. Jones C, Eddleston J, McCairn A, et al. Improving rehabilitation after critical illness through outpatient physiotherapy classes and essential amino acid supplement: a randomized controlled trial. *J Crit Care.* 2015;30(5):901–907.

102. Unützer J. IMPACT Intervention Manual. Unpublished manual; 1999.

103. Katon WJ, Von Korff M, Lin EH, et al. The Pathways Study: a randomized trial of collaborative care in patients with diabetes and depression. *Arch Gen Psychiatry.* 2004;61(10):1042–1049.

104. Martins RK, McNeil DW. Review of motivational interviewing in promoting health behaviors. *Clin Psychol Rev.* 2009;29(4):283–293.

105. Stevens RD, Dowdy DW, Michaels RK, et al. Neuromuscular dysfunction acquired in critical illness: a systematic review. *Intensive Care Med.* 2007;33(11):1876–1891.

106. Herridge MS, Cheung AM, Tansey CM, et al. One-year outcomes in survivors of the acute respiratory distress syndrome. *N Engl J Med.* 2003;348(8):683–693.

107. Thombs BD, Lawrence JW, Magyar-Russell G, et al. From survival to socialization: a longitudinal study of body image in survivors of severe burn injury. J Psychosom. Res. 2008;64(2):205–212.

108. Fauerbach JA, Heinberg LJ, Lawrence JW, et al. Effect of early body image dissatisfaction on subsequent psychological and physical adjustment after disfiguring injury. *Psychosom Med.* 2000;62(4):576–582.

109. Weinert CR, Gross CR, Kangas JR, et al. Health-related quality of life after acute lung injury. *Am J Respir Crit Care Med.* 1997;156(4 Pt 1):1120–1128.

110. Hopkins RO, Weaver LK, Chan KJ, et al. Quality of life, emotional, and cognitive function following acute respiratory distress syndrome. *J Int Neuropsychol Soc.* 2004;10(07):1005–1017.

111. Bienvenu OJ, Colantuoni E, Mendez-Tellez PA, et al. Depressive symptoms and impaired physical function after acute lung injury: a 2-year longitudinal study. *Am J Respir Crit Care Med.* 2012;185(5):517–524.

112. Prescott HC, Langa KM, Liu V, et al. Increased 1-year healthcare use in survivors of severe sepsis. *Am J Respir Crit Care Med.* 2014;190(1):62–69.

113. Liu V, Lei X, Prescott HC, et al. Hospital readmission and healthcare utilization following sepsis in community settings. *J Hosp Med.* 2014;9(8):502–507.

114. Unroe M, Kahn JM, Carson SS, et al. One-year trajectories of care and resource utilization for recipients of prolonged mechanical ventilation: a cohort study. *Ann Intern Med.* 2010;153(3):167–175.

115. McHugh LG, Milberg JA, Whitcomb ME, et al. Recovery of function in survivors of the acute respiratory distress syndrome. *Am J Respir Crit Care Med.* 1994;150(1):90–94.
116. Uchino BN, Cacioppo JT, Kiecolt-Glaser JK. The relationship between social support and physiological processes: a review with emphasis on underlying mechanisms and implications for health. *Psychol Bull.* 1996;119(3):488.
117. Tilburgs B, Nijkamp MD, Bakker EC, van der Hoeven H. The influence of social support on patients' quality of life after an intensive care unit discharge: a cross-sectional survey. *Intensive Crit Care Nurs.* 2015;31(6):336–342.
118. Borkovec T, Costello E. Efficacy of applied relaxation and cognitive-behavioral therapy in the treatment of generalized anxiety disorder. *J Consult Clin Psychol.* 1993;61(4):611.
119. Barlow DH, Gorman JM, Shear MK, et al. Cognitive-behavioral therapy, imipramine, or their combination for panic disorder: a randomized controlled trial. *JAMA.* 2000;283(19):2529–2536.
120. Sharp DM, Power KG, Simpson R, et al. Fluvoxamine, placebo, and cognitive behaviour therapy used alone and in combination in the treatment of panic disorder and agoraphobia. *J Anxiety Disord.* 1996;10(4):219–242.
121. Butler AC, Chapman JE, Forman EM, et al. The empirical status of cognitive-behavioral therapy: a review of meta-analyses. *Clin Psychol Rev.* 2006;26(1):17–31.
122. Beck AT, Sokol L, Clark DA, et al. A crossover study of focused cognitive therapy for panic disorder. *Am J Psychiatry.* 1992;149(6):778–783.
123. Beck JG, Stanley MA, Baldwin LE, et al. Comparison of cognitive therapy and relaxation training for panic disorder. *J Consult Clin Psychol.* 1994;62(4):818.

6

Prevention and Treatment of Posttraumatic Stress and Depressive Phenomena in Critical Illness Survivors

CHRISTINA JONES AND O. JOSEPH BIENVENU

INTRODUCTION

In the early 1990s little was known about recovery after critical illness. Patients were discharged from the intensive care unit (ICU) and followed up by their original admitting specialty, with no understanding of the added effects of critical illness. With the advent of ICU follow-up programs, either with questionnaires or in face-to-face outpatient clinic appointments, it became clear that patients and their families were struggling, both physically and psychologically, to recover from their illness. Gradually, over the past 20 years, there has been a shift in the opinion of ICU clinicians about the need to offer psychological help to patients and their families during the recovery period, as well as while the patient is still critically ill. Morbidity after an ICU stay can be high, with a wide range of psychological sequelae such as depression, anxiety,[1] and post-traumatic stress disorder (PTSD),[2] the symptoms of which can persist for months to years. This can have a massive impact on patients' quality of life, both during their recovery and over the years after their illness. A recent meta-analysis of studies on PTSD following critical illness found that the ICU risk factors for PTSD symptoms included benzodiazepine adminis-tration and post-ICU memories of frightening ICU experiences such as hallucinations or paranoid delusions.[3] Needing physical restraint in the ICU, which may be due to the agitation related to hyperactive delirium, and having a premorbid history of psychological problems have also been shown to increase the risk of post-ICU PTSD.[4,5] As noted in Chapter 4, severity of illness in the ICU was consistently *not* a predictor of PTSD.[3]

High levels of PTSD symptoms have been shown to be associated with worse quality of life after intensive care.[3] Similarly, in a study of anxiety and depression in recovering ICU patients, Kowalczyk and colleagues found that higher rates of these psychological problems were associated with adverse social and economic outcomes.[6]

In the BRAIN-ICU study, which was a prospective, multisite cohort study examining the recovery of medical/surgical ICU patients with respiratory failure or shock, Jackson and colleagues found that, at 3-month follow-up, 149 (37%) of 406 patients reported at least mild depression; at 12-month follow-up, 116 (33%) of 347 patients reported at least mild depression.[7] Standing out from other studies, only 7% of patients had symptom levels consistent with a possible diagnosis of PTSD at either follow-up point.

It should be remembered that psychological problems are also seen in relatives, particularly spouses, with high rates of anxiety, depression, and PTSD (see Chapter 8).[8] Importantly, relatives' mental health is relevant to the psychological outcomes of critical illness survivors, as they are the main caregivers when the patient goes home, so we will devote discussion to family members' mental health in Chapters 7 and 8.

PREVENTION OF PTSD AND DEPRESSION

Sedation

Higher sedative doses received in the ICU have been associated with worse PTSD symptoms, possibly through the mechanism of more

memories of frightening nightmares, hallucinations, and paranoid delusions, particularly in those patients with a premorbid history of psychological difficulties.[9] Such memories of hallucinations, nightmares,
or paranoid delusions, often of nurses trying to harm or kill them, are
described by patients as very vivid and realistic and can be difficult for
some individuals to accept as not being their real experience. These
memories are often the ones being relived in nightmares and flashbacks
as part of PTSD.[9] Daily interruption of sedation to assess patients' cognition and reduce the risk of oversedation is not only not harmful, it may
be beneficial to patients' long-term psychological outcomes.[10] Kress and
colleagues found, in the follow-up to their original study of sedation
breaks, that the intervention group had lower levels of PTSD symptoms
than in the control patients.[10]

In a single-center study, Strøm and colleagues examined the impact on
psychological recovery of a "no-sedation protocol," in which the investigators used opiates to ensure pain control (of course, opiates are also sedat-
ing).[11] Adult patients, mechanically ventilated for more than 24 hours,
were eligible for the study. The exclusion criteria were less than 18 years of
age, pregnancy, increased intracranial pressure, or a clinical need for sedation (for example, seizures or therapeutic hypothermia). The protocol aim
was for the intervention group to receive no propofol or benzodiazepine
sedation but rather to have bolus doses of morphine. If delirium was diagnosed, haloperidol was given. If an intervention patient was too distressed
at being awake, only 6 hours of non-morphine sedation could be given.
When a patient needed this three times they were given sedation, as in
the control group. The control group received normal continuous sedation and had daily interruption of their sedatives, propofol for the first
48 hours, changing to midazolam after this until the patient was ready to
be extubated. Control group patients were sedated to a Ramsay score of 3
to 4, which is fairly deep, as 3 is "Responsive to commands only" and 4 is
"Brisk response to light glabellar tap or loud auditory stimulus." In addition to sedation, the control patients were also given bolus doses of morphine. Psychological outcomes were assessed 2 years after randomization
using the Beck Depression Inventory II score, the State Anxiety Inventory,
and the Impact of Event Scale–Revised (IES-R) and the Post-Traumatic

Stress Syndrome 10-Questions Inventory (PTSS-10) to measure PTSD symptoms. The risk of long-term psychological problems was no different in the intervention group compared to the standard treatment group with propofol and midazolam sedation. Only one intervention patient, compared with three control patients, was classed as depressed using the Beck Depression Inventory. Both study groups had low IES-R scores, with only one intervention patient and two control patients with scores greater than 32. State anxiety scores were also low. Unfortunately, the generalizability of this study was limited since half of the randomized patients died before the 2-year follow-up assessment, and only half of the surviving patients were interviewed at this follow-up point.[11] In addition, the fact that patients in the control group were fairly deeply sedated (while now the sedation aim is often lighter) makes this a difficult study from which to generalize.

In a single-site randomized controlled trial (RCT) in a medical and surgical ICU, the rates of PTSD were compared in patients given light sedation or heavy sedation. The inclusion criteria were greater than 16 years of age, intubation, and mechanical ventilation for more than 12 hours. Patients were randomized to a midazolam-based sedation strategy with a target of either light sedation, Ramsay level 1–2 or deep sedation, Ramsay level 3-4. Morphine-based analgesia was also used in both groups. Standard protocols were used to wean patients off the ventilator. Psychological problems were the primary study endpoint, and PTSD, depression, and anxiety symptom scores were assessed at 4 weeks after ICU discharge. At 4-week follow-up, there were similar numbers of patients meeting diagnostic criteria for PTSD in both study groups (10% in the light sedation group vs. 9% in the deep sedation group). Anxiety and depression scores were also similar between the study groups. However, patients receiving deeper sedation had more disturbing memories of their ICU stay (18% vs. 4%) than did the light-sedation group.[12] While this is a negative study, the difference in recall of disturbing memories is interesting. As it is such memories that seem the basis of intrusive symptoms in PTSD, it is surprising that there was no difference between the study groups meeting diagnostic criteria for PTSD.

Corticosteroids

Sepsis, a massive systemic immune response to bacterial infection, is a common critical illness. Since inflammatory mediators can reduce the adrenal glands' responsiveness to adrenocorticotropic hormone, intensivists have investigated the usefulness of administering exogenous corticosteroids, given relatively low endogenous cortisol levels in septic patients. To the question of whether stress doses of corticosteroids improve survival, there is some evidence that stress doses of hydrocortisone prevent PTSD in patients with septic shock and in patients undergoing cardiac surgery.[13,14] The septic shock study was a prospective, randomized double-blind trial of the hemodynamic effects of stress doses of hydrocortisone in septic shock. Eleven control patients and 9 intervention patients were recruited to the study, and PTSD was diagnosed by psychiatrists using the Structured Clinical Interview for DSM-IV (SCID-IV; DSM-IV criteria). Seven of the 11 control patients, compared to only 1 out of the 9 intervention patients, developed PTSD ($p = .02$).[13]

The preventive effects of exogenous corticosteroid administration are being assessed in other patient populations as well; for example, Delahanty and colleagues investigated the impact of hydrocortisone in patients with acute physical trauma. Sixty-four patients were randomized, using a double-blind protocol, to receive either a 10-day course of hydrocortisone or placebo, started within 12 hours of the traumatic injury. The intervention patients reported fewer PTSD and depression symptoms and better health-related quality of life at 3-month follow-up than in the control patients.[15]

Intra-ICU psychological support

In Careggi Florence University Hospital in Italy, an early intra-ICU psychological intervention was established to prevent and treat psychological problems in trauma ICU patients.[16] The study was undertaken in the hospital's mixed ICU, which has 10 single-bed rooms. The nurse–patient ratio varied from 1:2 to 1:1 on some shifts, with a further one to three healthcare assistant nurses per shift. Up to two of the patients' relatives or friends had 24-hour access to the patients. Awake patients, if able to understand, and/ or their relatives were told about the clinical psychological service at ICU admission. The study started in April 2007, and the intervention aimed to prevent and treat the psychological impact of traumatic injury and critical illness; it was offered to patients, their families, and healthcare staff. A clinical psychologist was available on site from 12:00 to 16:00 and was then on call over the rest of the 24-hour period when needed. The service was staffed by three part-time clinical psychologists, with an annual cost of €30,000. Therapy was provided at the ICU bedside, and the patients were followed on the general wards after ICU discharge to ensure that further help was available if needed.

The psychological interventions provided by the clinical psychologists included educational interventions, counseling, stress management, psychological support, and information on coping strategies. Once awake and able to interact, patients received an average of five to six sessions with a clinical psychologist during their ICU stay. The interventions were all designed to manage anxiety, depression, fear, hopelessness, and helplessness. Cognitive and emotional restructuring formed the basis of the stress management intervention. The family interventions started while the patient was still sedated and aimed to promote family-centered decision-making and encourage relatives to choose appropriate interactions during their bedside visits. Family members were seen individually by the clinical psychologist.

There were 86 control patients and 123 intervention patients recruited to the study, and the two groups were similar in demographic and clinical characteristics. Clinically significant symptoms of anxiety and depression were assessed using a Hospital Anxiety and Depression Scale (HADS) subscale score greater than 11. PTSD symptoms were measured using the IES-R. The potential benefit of the service was tested in a before-and-after observational study. Patients from the intervention cohort had a lower prevalence of PTSD at 12-month follow-up as well as a trend toward a lower incidence of clinically significant anxiety and depression. In addition, a substantially lower percentage in the intervention cohort was on psychiatric medications at 12-month follow-up.[16]

A similar but much larger study in 24 U.K. ICUs has been set up to compare psychological outcomes of patients treated in ICUs in which the nurses have been trained in psychological interventions with outcomes of patients in ICUs staffed by nurses who have not received such training (the Provision Of Psychological support to People in Intensive care, or POPPI, Study). The intervention ICUs will have a training program for their nurses that aims to enable them to

- provide a calm, therapeutic environment for critically ill patients
- detect psychological distress in critically ill patients
- provide stress support sessions to their more distressed patients

The primary outcome of the study will be patient-reported PTSD symptom severity at 6 months and an economic analysis of the intervention. Secondary outcomes will be depression and health-related quality of life at 6 months. This study is currently ongoing.

Mobilization in the ICU

With the reduction in use of sedation in the ICU has come the possibility of more easily mobilizing and rehabilitating patients in the ICU, even while on mechanical ventilation. The research undertaken thus far suggests that early mobilization in critically ill patients improves physical function and can also reduce the duration of delirium by as much as 2 days.[17-19] Mobilization can be regarded as the primary nonpharmacological intervention to reduce the length of delirium in critically ill patients. It could be hypothesized that a reduction in the duration of delirium might translate to a lower risk of PTSD during recovery; unfortunately, as noted in Chapter 4, a number of studies have failed to show a *direct* relationship between delirium in the ICU and the later development of PTSD.[9,20,21] In addition, there are as yet no studies examining the psychological effects of early mobilization in ICU patients.

In other patient groups such as stroke survivors it has become clear that the immobility common after an acute stroke may increase negative mood symptoms. In the AVERT RCT the effect of very early mobilization after stroke (within 24 hours of the stroke) on levels of depression, anxiety, and irritability was evaluated. Seventy-one patients with confirmed stroke were recruited to the study, and at 7 days patients who were mobilized very early were less depressed than patients receiving standard care.[22]

Further research is needed to understand the impact of early mobilization on ICU patients' psychological recovery.

TREATMENT OF POSTTRAUMATIC STRESS AND DEPRESSIVE PHENOMENA

Rehabilitation programs

As noted in Chapter 5, recent studies have tried to address the physical, cognitive, and psychological rehabilitation needs of patients recovering from critical illness. A number of interventions have been designed and tested to aid in that recovery. In an RCT of rehabilitation following critical illness, Jones and colleagues tested a 6-week manualized rehabilitation program, the ICU Recovery Manual.[23] The manual contained self-directed exercises, information about the aftereffects of critical illness, and psychological advice about anxiety, depression, and PTSD. The content of the ICU Recovery Manual was based around solutions to the many problems reported by 5 years' worth of ICU outpatient clinic patients, as well as patients and families attending the ICU support group at Whiston Hospital, UK. The draft manual was piloted on 20 critical illness survivors before the study began. At 2-month follow-up, the intervention was associated with lower levels of depression and PTSD-related symptoms as assessed using the IES.[23] At 6-month follow-up, the rate of depression in the two study groups was very similar: 10% in the patients receiving the ICU Recovery Manual and 12% in control patients. When a cut-off score of ≥19 on the IES was applied there was no difference in clinically significant PTSD symptoms between the study groups at 6 months.[23]

Subsequently, the Program of Enhanced Physiotherapy & Structured Exercise (PEPSE) was developed. This program involves the patient taking part in three 1-hour physiotherapist-led exercise sessions per week while in the hospital, one 1-hour supervised outpatient session after the patient is discharged home, and two home exercise sessions per week for 6 weeks. In a nonrandomized pilot study, 38 critical illness survivors who completed the program had significant reductions in anxiety and depression.[24]

We recently conducted an RCT of PEPSE, with or without a glutamine and essential amino acid (GEEA) supplement drink given in between meals. The inclusion criteria were that patients should be 45 years or older, have a combined ICU and pre-ICU stay of 5 days or more, and be able to engage in the physiotherapy program. The study had a 2 × 2 factorial design, with the nutritional supplement double-blinded and the physiotherapy single-blinded at the follow-up assessment. All study patients received the updated ICU Recovery Manual.[23] The primary study endpoint was the 6-Minute Walk Test (6MWT), and the secondary outcomes were anxiety and depression measured using the HADS at 3 months. The nutritional intervention GEAA and a similar tasting low-calorie control supplement were supplied as identical powder mixtures in sachets and made up by the patients as needed by mixing with water or juice, if the palpability was a problem. The results of the study demonstrated a significant reduction in anxiety in both PEPSE study arms, as well as a reduction in depression in the GEAA supplement/PEPSE study arm.[25] The positive effect of the intervention on anxiety and depression may, in part, be due to fact that the patients receiving PEPSE were able to share their experiences with other patients in the outpatient exercise class, thus normalizing their experience. In addition, there is some research suggesting a positive impact of nutrition on depression.[26]

There are recognized positive psychological benefits of exercise on mood. A review of general research on the psychological impact of exercise showed that, in the main, exercise and physical activity are associated with better health outcomes, improved quality of life, and improvements in mood states, such as anxiety and depression.[27] The review was wide-ranging and included cross-sectional studies, longitudinal studies, and randomized clinical trials. The study groups included individuals with physical conditions, such as obesity, cancer, cardiovascular disease, and sexual dysfunction. In addition, studies looking at the impact of exercise on depression and other mood states were included. The studies included in the review covered a wide range of ethnicities, and sex and age groups, making it applicable to a number of populations. One of the major limitations was the limited sample sizes of many of the RCTs and short follow-up periods.

The scarcity of RCTs examining the impact of exercise programs on depression and anxiety in recovering ICU patients, except for the ones discussed here, would support the need for further research.

ICU diaries

Since the 1980s, nurses have kept ICU diaries in Scandinavia. Originally, these were simply written diaries, but they evolved into photo diaries, which combine text with photographs taken at points of change in the patients' ICU stay.[28] ICU diaries are now being adopted worldwide to help patients come to terms with their critical illness experience (see the adoption map on www.icu-diary.org). Most ICUs introducing diaries now use the model of daily entries by both healthcare professionals, predominately bedside nurses, and relatives and friends. Photographs are taken at the start of the diary and at points of change in the patients' condition or treatment, for example, following the insertion of a tracheostomy. The healthcare staff entries should all be written in everyday language, with any technical terms explained in the text, so that a patient is able to understand the contents of the diary without the need to look up medical terms (although brief glossaries can be useful supplements). The photographs should be taken so that the patient is recognizable and should include healthcare staff and relatives where feasible. In the United Kingdom a photocopy of the diary is entered into the medical notes, as the diary is viewed as partly a medical document. Diaries are normally given to patients when they feel ready for them; this may be in the ICU, on the general wards, or in an outpatient clinic after hospital discharge. In cases in which the patient dies in the hospital, many relatives usually want to receive the diary. In the experience of the first author (CJ) of this chapter, some of the most moving diary entries are written by relatives and friends saying goodbye to dying patients (see Figure 6.1). Some relatives actually put the diary in the coffin with the deceased patient as a collection of all their goodbyes.

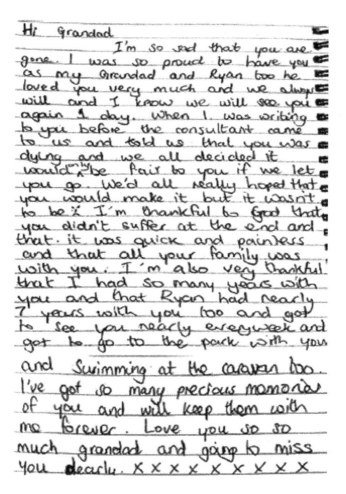

Figure 6.1. Farewell to a beloved grandfather (from Jones C. Farewell to a beloved grandfather. *Intensive Care Medicine* 2013;39[7]:1321[53]).

A Danish study examined how patients felt about their ICU diaries; the results indicated that diaries helped patients recognize the presence of the nurses during their ICU stays, which they probably would not remember; patients also reported that the diary was a source of comfort, encouragement, and hope.[29] The same researchers compared the use of hospital records or an ICU diary to help patients to understand their illness; patients felt that the diary gave them a more comprehensive explanation of their time in the ICU.[30] Figures 6.2, 6.3, 6.4, and 6.5, and Boxes 6.1 and 6.2 illustrate components of an ICU diary, modeled at Johns Hopkins after those at Whiston Hospital, UK, and other centers (see www.icu-diary.org).

Several studies have examined the impact of ICU diaries on patients' psychological recovery after they leave the hospital. A small RCT ($n = 36$)

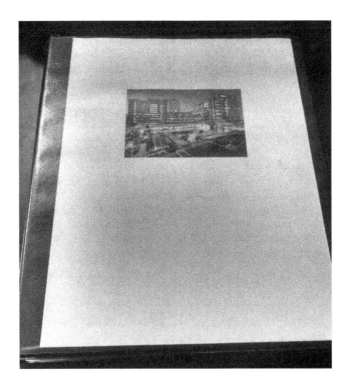

Figure 6.2. A three-ring binder, containing a patient's ICU diary, placed outside the patient's room in the Johns Hopkins Hospital Medical ICU.

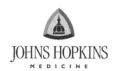

JOHNS HOPKINS
M E D I C I N E

PATIENT DIARIES: INFORMATION FOR PATIENTS AND RELATIVES

Patients who have had a stay in the intensive care unit (ICU) often have little or no memory of it. Their memory for this time can be affected by the illness itself or the sedative drugs we give to our patients to keep them comfortable and safe. Patients may also remember nightmares or hallucinations from this time that can be very frightening.

Although doctors and nurses explain why patients were admitted to the ICU, patients and family members often forget what we have told them. Research has suggested that patients can become stressed and anxious when they do not understand what has been wrong with them. To help patients and family members understand a patient's illness and ICU stay, the staff have introduced patient diaries. ICU diaries have been shown to reduce stress in patients and family members in the months after an ICU stay.

The nurses make daily diary entries to explain what has brought the patient to the ICU, what is wrong, and how things are progressing. Some patients may also have their photograph taken for their diary.

We encourage loved ones to write in the diary, to pass on your messages to the patient or to tell them news from home that they would like to hear. When writing in the diary, please avoid using any language that could cause offense to the patient or others who may read the diary afterwards.

The diary will be kept outside the patient's ICU room; you just need to ask the nurse looking after your relative if you would like to make a diary entry.

When our patients are well enough and are ready for transfer to a general ward, we go through the diaries with them, if possible. Once patients are well enough to look after their diary, they are allowed to keep them if they wish.

Please remember that the diary is hospital property until handed over to the patient after he or she signs a consent form.

Diaries must not be taken away by family members.

If you have any questions about patient diaries, please do not hesitate to ask the nurse looking after your relative.

Figure 6.3. ICU diary information for patients and relatives.

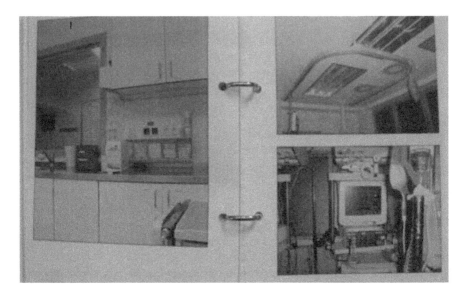

Figure 6.4. Photographs of an ICU room from the patient's perspective, for later orientation.

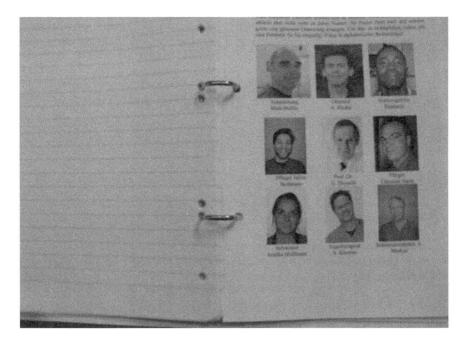

Figure 6.5. Photographs of the treating team for later orientation.

Box 6.1 EXAMPLE (HAND-WRITTEN) ENTRIES IN AN ICU DIARY

Initial entry (for Patient 1):

Today you came to the emergency department (ED) by ambulance with your son and daughter. They called 911 at home after you fell down and were not able to talk to them. Your speech was slurred in the ED, and you weren't able to move your legs. You started having trouble breathing and had a seizure, so the doctors put a breathing tube through your mouth into your lungs so you could breathe. You had a CT scan of your head and chest to make sure you didn't have a stroke. You also were transferred to the ICU where we put in a central line into your neck for medications. After about 12 hours, you became very upset and agitated, and we had to give you medicine to relax. Your son and two daughters stayed with you all day. Your breathing improved, and we were able to remove the breathing tube. You became even more agitated and pulled at your Foley catheter that was draining your urine. We gave you some medicine and you started to wake up and follow directions. Your daughter stayed with you all night long.

Follow-up (daily) entry (for Patient 2):

Today was a good day for you. You still have the breathing tube in, but you are more alert and able to squeeze my hand when I ask you to. Physical therapy came to see you today, and you were able to push the pedals of the bed bike for 20 minutes while lying in your hospital bed. Your blood pressure has improved and is stable now, and your temperature has been normal. You still have two peripheral IV lines in your right and left arms and a Foley catheter in your penis to drain your urine. Your son came by to visit today and stayed all afternoon. You began breathing too fast when we changed the ventilator to let you breathe more on your own, so we had to rest you after an hour. Tomorrow the plan is to try a ventilator weaning trial again to help strengthen your lungs.

Box 6.2 DIARY GLOSSARY FOR PATIENTS AND FAMILY MEMBERS

Arterial line: Many ICU patients have an arterial line, usually in the wrist. This is connected to a monitor and shows your blood pressure. Arterial lines also allow us to take blood samples.

Bronchoscope: This procedure is carried out using a fiber-optic camera device. The scope is passed through your breathing tube into the air passages leading to the lungs, allowing the doctor to see into the airways of the lungs, wash out secretions, and sometimes take biopsies.

Central line or central venous line: Most ICU patients will have one of these lines; they are usually put in the neck or groin. They have lots of ports allowing different drugs to be given at the same time. They are linked to the monitor and are sometimes kept in when you go to a regular hospital ward.

CPAP/BiPAP: This gives extra help with breathing and is connected to an endotracheal tube or tracheostomy. The patient is doing all the breathing, and the continuous positive airway pressure (CPAP) or bi-level positive airway pressure (BiPAP) helps keep the airways open.

CPAP/BiPAP face mask: This is a tight-fitting face mask that gives extra help with breathing by opening the airways.

Endotracheal tube: This is a tube that goes into the windpipe through the mouth and then is connected to the ventilator for oxygen.

Flexiseal: This is a rectal tube to collect loose stools (diarrhea).

Foley catheter: This is a tube that drains the bladder by gravity—it is passed through the urethra, and the urine gathers in a waterproof box or bag.

Nasal (nose) cannula: This is a way of giving oxygen through tubes that fit into the nostrils.

Nasogastric (NG) tube: This is a tube that passes into the stomach from one side of your nose. Many ICU patients have one of these. It is used to drain the stomach if you are vomiting or to give food and medicines.

> **Nebulizer:** This makes medicine into a mist and helps loosen thick phlegm and open the airways.
>
> **Tracheostomy:** This is when a tube is inserted into the windpipe through an incision in the skin of the neck. It needs a small operation and usually replaces the endotracheal tube, and it can be more comfortable than an endotracheal tube when the sedation is turned off.
>
> **Ventilator:** This is also known as a breathing machine; it does the breathing for you.

examined the effect of receiving a diary on anxiety and depression and found that those who received a diary had lower levels of both these symptoms.[31] A second, multi-country European RCT examined the effect of ICU diaries on the incidence of first-onset PTSD. Twelve ICUs in six European countries—the UK, Sweden, Norway, Denmark, Italy, and Portugal—recruited patients to the study. The ICUs in Italy and Portugal were not already using diaries but were very keen to join the study, so they had a 3-month lead-in to the study, to allow the diaries to become embedded before starting patient recruitment. Patients with an ICU stay of more than 72 hours were recruited to the study. The intervention patients received their diary at 1 month following ICU discharge, and the final assessment of the development of acute PTSD was made at 3 months. Control patients were able to receive their diary after they had completed their 3-month follow-up questionnaires. A total of 352 patients completed the 3-month follow-up. The study results showed that the intervention group had a reduced prevalence of new-onset PTSD (due to the ICU experience), 5%, compared to 13% for the controls.[32] The effect was most noticeable in those patients with high levels of PTSD symptoms at the 1-month time point, assessed just prior to being offered the diary. These patients with high levels of PTSD symptoms had a significant fall in the level of PTSD symptoms by the 3-month follow-up. Intervention patients were asked to provide feedback on their experience of receiving a diary.

The majority were very positive about their diary, and most had read it a median of three times (range, 0 to 20); only one patient had not read the diary. Eighty-four percent of patients reported that other people had read their diary, with family members being the most common (100%), followed by friends (36%), work colleagues (5%), and other healthcare staff, such as their general practitioner (4%). When asked to comment on what they felt helped most, only two (1.4%) patients mentioned their meeting with the nurse to go through the diary; 49% felt the written entries in the diary were most helpful; 36% thought it was the writing and photographs together, and 15% thought the photographs helped most. A subanalysis of two study ICUs with data on the levels of PTSD symptoms in relatives showed lower levels in families when the patient was in the diary intervention group.[33]

A third study, from France, using a before-and-after cohort design, also examined the effect of diaries, written by staff and relatives, on mental health outcomes. The first entry in the diary was standardized and included an explanation of why the diary was being written, as well as a chart of the ICU staff with their photographs. Photographs of an empty ICU room, of the entrance to the ICU, and of the patient's room from the patient's perspective were also entered in the diary (with written explanations). Then a summary of the patient's history before ICU admission was entered. Depending on the machines used to treat the patient, photographs of the ventilator and/or dialysis machines were added. No patient photographs were taken. The diary was then maintained by the family and ICU staff. The study showed that the rate of severe PTSD symptoms at 12 months post-ICU was lower in those patients who received a diary (pre-diary period 35%, diary period 21%, and post-diary period 30%).[34] The study also assessed PTSD symptoms in relatives at 12 months post-ICU, and the rate of high levels of symptoms varied significantly across the study periods (pre-diary period 80%, diary period 31.7%, and post-diary period 67.6%).

Despite the apparent beneficial effects of ICU diaries, their routine use appears relatively uncommon in North America, apparently for fear of lawsuits. In addition, some authors have noted that ICU diary contents vary quite a bit across centers, and the mechanism of their apparent benefit remains unclear.[35] Ullman and colleagues recently conducted a Cochrane systematic review and discouraged the routine use of ICU diaries.[35] We respectfully disagree with those authors. Specifically, the reviews' authors did not feel that the main outcome measure (of new-onset PTSD) in the study by Jones and colleagues[32] had been validated sufficiently for inclusion in the review; however, we note that the authors accepted a continuous PTSD symptom measure (the PTSS-14)[36] that had been validated *against* the main outcome measure in the study (the PTSD Diagnostic Scale).[32] Given the overall apparent benefit, the low cost, and the lack of harm from ICU diaries, we *do* encourage their routine use, as well as further study.

Support groups and group meetings

In the United Kingdom there has been a growth in ICU support groups for both patients and relatives to talk about their experience of critical illness and the ICU.[37,38] Jones and her colleagues at Whiston Hospital found that it was important not to use a room in the hospital to meet because it brought up unwanted reminders of the critical illness. The support group met instead in a private side room in a local pub, with the patients and relatives allowed to buy themselves a beer but the staff going dry![37] This meeting place encourage a relaxed atmosphere and open access for patients and their families. They felt able to share their ICU experiences, recovery advice, and worries. ICU staff were available to answer any medical questions but otherwise allowed the discussion to proceed unhindered. The support group ran for 5 years, but it took a lot of commitment from the staff member who organized it (CJ) and was eventually dropped because of her PhD commitments.

Peskett and Gibb have written about setting up their first local support group and the founding of their charity, ICUsteps (see Chapter 1).[38] Drop-in sessions were set up that allowed patients and relatives to share their experiences with others who had personal experience with the

ICU. Individuals attending the drop-in sessions felt that the support was needed and that they benefited through sharing their experiences with others who had been through critical illness themselves. The structure of ICUsteps support groups is different from that for the Whiston Hospital patients and families. Instead of the organization of the drop-in sessions falling on one nurse, a cohort of patients and relatives volunteer to help. This makes the drop-in meetings much more sustainable. ICUsteps, with the UK Intensive Care Society Foundation, have produced a guide for setting up patient and family support groups, which can be downloaded as a pdf file.[39] There are now 20 ICUsteps-style support groups running in the United Kingdom.

In a recent Swedish descriptive intervention-based study examining the impact of group meetings for partners of surviving ICU patients, two group sessions, lasting 2 hours, were held at monthly intervals, and the participants kept notes about their feelings of taking part in the meetings. To expand the understanding of the impact of these sessions, six of the partners were interviewed in depth.[40] Three categories were identified by content analysis of the notes and interviews: (1) emotional impact—there was a feeling of togetherness and gratitude for shared worries; (2) confirmation of their experience through reflection; (3) the meeting design was supported, and participants' recommended that the groups should be continued.[40] Results from parallel group sessions with recovering ICU patients have been analyzed and as of this writing are soon to be published.

Social support has been shown to be one of most important factors in predicting well-being across a wide range of ages. The level of social support given to individuals is an important factor in successfully overcoming life stress. Social support is a major factor in preventing negative emotional phenomena such as depression.[41] While family members would normally be a major source of social support to the patient, in a traumatic situation such as critical illness, relatives can be too distressed to provide such support. The provision of peer support through drop-in sessions and group meetings may fill the gap until the family coping strategies are able to work again.

Currently, there are no studies examining the impact of patient and family support groups on psychological recovery. Hopefully, now that the number of support groups using the ICUsteps' model is increasing, such research can begin to be planned.

Psychological therapies after the ICU

Psychological therapies provided by a licensed counselor, social worker, clinical psychologist, or psychiatrist are expensive and should perhaps be targeted to those patients with the greatest need. The UK National Institute of Clinical Excellence has published a number of guidelines on the recognition and treatment of anxiety,[42] depression,[43] and PTSD.[44] The backbone of all of the guidelines is the importance of appropriate assessment in high-risk groups to ensure prompt referrals for treatment. For those with low symptom levels, a "watch and wait" approach is recommended, with a provision for reassessment later in recovery to ensure there has not been an increase in symptoms. The routine use of short screening tools such as the PTSS-14[45] or the IES-R[46] for PTSD-related symptoms and the HADS[47] may facilitate the recognition of ICU survivors with high levels of PTSD, anxiety, and depression symptoms.

In the United Kingdom an ICU nurse–led counseling service was benchmarked against a cancer counseling service and a community-based service. The two ICU nurses running the service had both retrained as counselors but could fall back on their ICU nursing experience when required. ICU patients attending this service were shown in the study to have the most severe initial symptoms, compared to the cancer and community-based services. Despite the initial severity of the symptoms the majority of the ICU patients were nonsymptomatic at the end of counseling.[48] Former ICU patients have reported common themes during counseling: trying to make sense of what happened in the ICU, coming to terms with physical changes, and coping with distressing flashbacks or nightmares.[48,49] Therapies used in the service included trauma-focused cognitive-behavioral therapy (CBT), to facilitate learning of new skills to help process thoughts and feelings related to the traumatic memories from ICU; manage and resolve distressing thoughts, feelings, and behaviors; and enhance safety, growth, and family communication. Eye movement desensitization and reprocessing (EMDR) was also used to help patients reduce the long-lasting effects of distressing memories by developing more adaptive coping mechanisms. The therapy uses an eight-phase approach that includes having the patient recall distressing images while receiving one of several types of bilateral sensory input, such as side-to-side eye movements. An important first step is to reinforce a safe place; this may be a place from childhood that the patient can easily access in the mind which makes them feel safe, or it may simply involve the patient imagining sitting in his or her garden in the sun and feeling relaxed. For some patients who have had a traumatic or deprived childhood this is not an easy task, and it becomes necessary to use the therapeutic relationship to instill a feeling of safety in the counseling room. Hypnotherapy can be useful to help reinforce the safe place, as hypnosis involves the individual experiencing deep relaxation and focusing on appropriate suggestions made by the therapist. Individual hypnotherapy scripts can be recorded by the therapist for the patient to take home on CD and use there to reinforce their safe place and gain some relaxation. The ability of the patient to go to his or her safe place easily is important before EMDR can be commenced on any intrusive memories, as in that work the therapist will instruct the patient to go to the safe place if the patient suddenly feels overwhelmed by memories.

Patients may initially belittle their frightening memories of nightmares, paranoid delusions, and hallucinations in the ICU, saying they are silly or that the therapist will think they are crazy if they speak about them.[2,49] Being able to normalize these experiences and tell patients that they are common, but still have patients accept their memories as their lived experience, is an important first step to moving on. These memories will always be there; the aim of therapy is not to remove them but to help take away their power to run the patients' lives and stopping them from sleeping properly, socializing, returning for medical appointments, or engaging in family life. Such intrusive memories appear to be happening in the "here and now," and with therapy, the frequency, vividness, distress, and seeming now-ness fades.[50]

As a therapist, Dr. Jones has accompanied patients to the anesthesia room prior to surgery to ground patients in reality and help them stay in their safe place, as anesthesia is a powerful stressor for a small number of patients.

In depression, intrusive memories can still be present, but the distress and sensory quality are lower than in PTSD. Similarly, the proportion of sensory words in the narrative describing the intrusive memories is lower among depressed patients compared to those with PTSD.[51] Intrusive memories in PTSD have more sensory content and fewer time markers, which would fit with the here-and-now quality of such memories. Basic sensory processes contribute to the intrusiveness of remembering in PTSD, but not in depression.[51]

Traditional forms of CBT for depression do not normally target negative intrusive memories. A small number of studies have produced evidence for the use of imaginal exposure and re-scripting of imagery to reduce their impact in depression. In trauma-focused CBT, techniques such as cognitive restructuring and behavioral experiments are used to change maladaptive appraisals of the trauma and intrusive re-experiencing. In a study looking at both computer-based and therapist-delivered cognitive restructuring and psychoeducation, there were significant reductions in both study groups in depression, memory intrusiveness, and negative appraisals.[52]

CONCLUSIONS

Patients recovering from critical illness can be left with significant psychological problems that have a profound effect on their quality of life. As yet, studies on prevention of PTSD and/or depression are in their infancy. However, providing ICU diaries for as many patients as possible is a simple and cost-effective way of helping patients come to terms with their ICU experience. Also, multimodal rehabilitation strategies that can improve psychological recovery are beginning to be established. Recognizing those patients needing further help through routine psychological screening during follow-up and having a structured pathway for rehabilitation is the first step in returning patients to as normal a life as possible.

REFERENCES

1. Jones C, Griffiths RD, Macmillan RR, Palmer TEA. Psychological problems occurring after intensive care. *Br J Intensive Care*. 1994;2:46–53.
2. Jones C, Humphris GH, Griffiths RD. Psychological morbidity following critical illness—the rationale for care after intensive care. *Clin Intensive Care*. 1998;9:199–205.
3. Parker AM, Sricharoenchai T, Raparla S, Schneck KW, Bienvenu OJ, Needham DM. Posttraumatic stress disorder in critical illness survivors: a meta-analysis. *Crit Care Med*. 2015;43(5):1121–1129.
4. Jones C, Griffiths RD. Patient and caregiver counselling after the intensive care unit: what are the needs and how should they be met? *Curr Opin Crit Care*. 2007;13:503–507.
5. Davydow DS, Gifford JM, Desai SV, Needham DM, Bienvenu OJ. Posttraumatic stress disorder in general intensive care unit survivors: a systematic review. *Gen Hosp Psychiatry*. 2008;30(5):421–434.
6. Kowalczyk M, Nestrorowicz A, Fijalkowska A, Kwiatisz-Muc M. Emotional sequelae among survivors of critical illness: a long-term retrospective study. *Eur J Anaesthesiol*. 2013;30(3):111–118.
7. Jackson JC, Pandharipande PP, Girard TD, et al. Depression, post-traumatic stress disorder, and functional disability in survivors of critical illness in the BRAIN-ICU study: a longitudinal cohort study. *Lancet Respir Med*. 2014;2(5):369–379.
8. Schmidt M, Azoulay E. Having a loved one in ICU: the forgotten family. *Curr Opin Crit Care*. 2012;18(5):540–547.
9. Jones C, Backman C, Capuzzo M, Flaatten H, Rylander C, Griffiths RD. Precipitants of post-traumatic stress disorder following intensive care: a hypothesis generating study of diversity in care. *Intensive Care Med*. 2007;33(6):978–985.
10. Kress JP, Gehlbach B, Lacy M, Pliskin N, Pohlman AS, Hall JB. The long-term psychological effects of daily sedative interruption on critically ill patients. *Am J Respir Crit Care Med*. 2003;168(12):1457–1461.
11. Strøm T, Stylsvig M, Toft P. Long-term psychological effects of a no-sedation protocol in critically ill patients. *Crit Care*. 2011;15(6):R293.
12. Treggiari MM, Romand JA, Yanez ND, Deem SA, Goldberg J, Hudson L, Heidegger CP. Randomized trial of light versus deep sedation on mental health after critical illness. *Crit Care Med*. 2009;37(9):2527–2534.
13. Schelling G, Briegel J, Roozendaal B, Stoll C, Rothenhäusler HB, Kapfhammer HP. The effect of stress doses of hydrocortisone during septic shock on posttraumatic stress disorder in survivors. *Biol Psychiatry*. 2001;50(12):978–985.

14. Schelling G. Post-traumatic stress disorder in somatic disease: lessons from critically ill patients. *Prog Brain Res.* 2008;167:229–237.

15. Delahanty DL, Gabert-Quillen C, Ostrowski SA, et al. The efficacy of initial hydrocortisone administration at preventing posttraumatic distress in adult trauma patients: a randomized trial. *CNS Spectr.* 2013;18(2):103–11113.

16. Peris A, Bonizzoli M, Iozzelli D, et al. Early intra-intensive care unit psychological intervention promotes recovery from post traumatic stress disorders, anxiety and depression symptoms in critically ill patients. *Crit Care.* 2011;15(1):R41.

17. Schweickert WD, Pohlman MC, Pohlman AS et al. Early physical and occupational therapy in mechanically ventilated, critically ill patients: a randomised controlled trial. *Lancet.* 2009;373(9678):1874–1882.

18. Needham DM, Korupolu R, Zanni JM, et al. Early physical medicine and rehabilitation for patients with acute respiratory failure: a quality improvement project. *Arch Phys Med Rehabil.* 2010;91(4):536–542.

19. Needham DM, Korupolu R. Rehabilitation quality improvement in an intensive care unit setting: implementation of a quality improvement model. *Top Stroke Rehabil.* 2010;17(4):271–281.

20. Girard TD, Shintani AK, Jackson JC, et al. Risk factors for post-traumatic stress disorder symptoms following critical illness requiring mechanical ventilation: a prospective cohort study. *Crit Care.* 2007;11:R28.

21. Bienvenu OJ, Gellar J, Althouse BM, et al. Post-traumatic stress disorder symptoms after acute lung injury: a 2-year prospective longitudinal study. *Psychol Med.* 2013;43(12):2657–2671.

22. Cumming TB, Collier JM, Thrift AG, Bernhardt J. The effect of very early mobilization after stroke on psychological well-being. *J Rehabil Med.* 2008;40(8):609–614.

23. Jones C, Skirrow P, Griffiths RD, et al. Rehabilitation after critical illness: a randomized, controlled trial. *Crit Care Med.* 2003;31(10):2456–2461.

24. McWilliams DJ, Atkinson D, Carter A. Feasibility and impact of a structured, exercise-based rehabilitation programme for intensive care survivors. *Physiother Theory Pract.* 2009;25(8):566–571.

25. Jones C, Eddleston J, McCairn A, et al. Improving rehabilitation after critical illness through outpatient physiotherapy classes and essential amino acid supplement: a randomized controlled trial. *J Crit Care.* 2015;30(7):901–907.

26. Lakhan SE, Vieira KF. Nutritional therapies for mental disorders *Nutr J.* 2008;7:2. doi: 10.1186/1475-2891-7-2

27. Penedo FJ, Dahn JR. Exercise and well-being: a review of mental and physical health benefits associated with physical activity. *Curr Opin Psychiatry.* 2005;18(2):189–193.

28. Bäckman C, Jones C. Implementing a diary programme in your ICU. *ICU Manage.* 2011;11(3):10–16.

29. Egerod I, Christensen D. Analysis of patient diaries in Danish ICUs: a narrative approach. *Intensive Crit Care Nurs.* 2009;25(5):268–277.

30. Egerod I, Christensen D. A comparative study of ICU patients diaries vs hospital charts. *Qual Health Res.* 2010;22(10):1446–1456.

31. Knowles RE, Tarrier N. Evaluation of the effect of prospective patient diaries on emotional well-being in intensive care unit survivors: a randomised control trial. *Crit Care Med.* 2009;37(1):184–191.

32. Jones C, Bäckman C, Capuzzo M, et al. Intensive care diaries reduce new onset PTSD following critical illness: a randomised, controlled trial. *Crit Care.* 2010;14(5):R168.

33. Jones C, Bäckman C, Griffith C. Intensive care diaries reduce PTSD-related symptoms in relatives following critical illness. *Am J Crit Care.* 2012;21(3):172–176.

34. Garrouste-Orgeas M, Coquet I, Périer A, et al. Impact of an intensive care unit diary on psychological distress in patients and relatives. *Crit Care Med.* 2012;40(7):2033–2040.

35. Aitken LM, Rattray J, Hull A, Kenardy JA, Le Broque R, Ullman AJ. The use of diaries in psychological recovery from intensive care. *Crit Care.* 2013;17(6):253.

36. Ullman AJ, Aitken LM, Rattray J, et al. Diaries for recovery from critical illness. *Cochrane Database Syst Rev.* 2014;12:CD010468.

37. Jones C, Macmillan RR, Griffiths RD. Providing psychological support to patients after critical illness. *Clin Intensive Care.* 1994;5(4):176–179.

38. Peskett M, Gibb P. Developing and setting up a patient and relative intensive care support group. *Nurs Crit Care.* 2009;14(1):4–10.

39. ICU Steps. Local support groups. http://icusteps.org/support. Accessed April 21, 2016.

40. Ahlberg M, Bäckman C, Jones C, Walther S, Frisman GH. Moving on in life after intensive care—partners' experience of group communication. *Nurs Crit Care.* 2015;20(5):256–263.

41. Russell DW, Cutrona CE. Social support, stress, and depressive symptoms among the elderly: test of a process model. *Psychol Aging.* 1991;6(2):190–201.

42. Generalised anxiety disorder and panic disorder in adults: management. https://www.nice.org.uk/guidance/cg113. Accessed April 21, 2016.

43. Depression in adults: recognition and management. https://www.nice.org.uk/guidance/cg90. Accessed April 21, 2016.

44. Post-traumatic stress disorder: management. https://www.nice.org.uk/guidance/cg26. Accessed April 21, 2016.

45. Twigg E, Humphris G, Jones C, Bramwell R, Griffiths RD. Use of a screening questionnaire for post-traumatic stress disorder (PTSD) on a sample of UK ICU patients. *Acta Anaesthesiol Scand.* 2008;52(2):202–208.

46. Bienvenu OJ, Williams JB, Yang A, Hopkins RO, Needham DM. Posttraumatic stress disorder in survivors of acute lung injury: evaluating the Impact of Event Scale-Revised. *Chest.* 2013;144(1):24–31.

47. Zigmond AS, Snaith RP. The Hospital Anxiety and Depression Scale. *Acta Psychiatr Scand.* 1983;67(6):361–370.

48. Jones C, Hall S, Jackson S. Benchmarking a nurse-led ICU counselling initiative. *Nurs Times.* 2008;104(38):32–34.

49. Barnett L. Intensive care: an existential perspective. *Therapy Today.* 2006;17(5):10–15.

50. Hackmann A, Ehlers A, Speckens A, Clark DM. Characteristics and content of intrusive memories in PTSD and their changes with treatment. *J Trauma Stress.* 2004;17(3):231–240.

51. Parry L, O'Kearney R. A comparison of the quality of intrusive memories in post-traumatic stress disorder and depression. *Memory*. 2014;22(4):404–425.

52. Newby JM, Lang T, Werner-Seidler, Holmes E, Moulds ML. Alleviating distressing intrusive memories in depression: A comparison between computerised cognitive bias modification and cognitive behavioural education *Behav Res Ther*. 2014;56(100):60–67.

53. Jones C. Farewell to a beloved grandfather. *Intensive Care Med*. 2013;39(7):1321.

7

Supporting Pediatric Patients and Their Families during and after Intensive Care Treatment

GILLIAN COLVILLE

INTRODUCTION

As the literature on the physical and psychological sequelae of critical illness mounts, clinicians and researchers working in this field are increasingly coming to appreciate the extent to which survivors continue to be affected by their traumatic experiences during and after their treatment in the intensive care unit (ICU). Greater awareness of the ways in which relatives are also affected emotionally has led to recommendations that units give greater consideration to the needs of family members and that their emotional status should also be monitored after discharge.

The focus of most of the recent calls for the development of dedicated services to address psychological problems in patients and families has been on adult patients,[1] reflecting the fact that most intensive care patients are adults. However, there is also compelling evidence that *pediatric* intensive care patients and their family members are adversely affected psychologically. Indeed, there are at least two good reasons to suppose that the relatives of pediatric patients might actually be at *increased* risk for distress as compared with relatives of adult ICU patients. The relative infrequency of pediatric ICU (PICU) admissions and the consequent tendency for critical care services to be centralized in the interests of patient safety mean that families often live a considerable distance from the hospital where their child is being treated. This increases the strain on families, both in terms of time spent traveling back and forth and in terms of time away from other family members. Second, while it is estimated that the proportion of relatives who find themselves in the role of caregiver after an adult ICU admission is approximately 50%,[2] it is clear that a parent is in this role in 100% of cases following a PICU admission.

In this chapter I will attempt to show how the observations and recommendations in the adult ICU literature are relevant to the provision of services for pediatric intensive care patients and their families. In doing so, I will refer to two relevant models of service currently in use in pediatric settings, draw on the research in this field, and illustrate with clinical examples. I will suggest some ways in which health professionals can support families in this difficult situation.

Davidson, a pioneer in drawing attention to the psychological impact of the ICU,[3] has spearheaded the recent work of the Society of Critical Care Medicine (SCCM) task force on what has come to be termed *post–intensive care syndrome* (PICS, or PICS-F when referring to its occurrence in family members). This comprises a cluster of psychological complications reported in relation to experiences during, and subsequent to, intensive care admission. These commonly include anxiety, depression, and posttraumatic stress and, post-discharge, may relate to loss of function or disfigurement for patients and increased burden of care for relatives. Davidson makes an impassioned plea for properly structured services to address these manifestations of distress,[4] arguing that this is a serious public health issue and, as such, much more than "just a nice thing to do."[5] While the terms *PICS* and *PICS-F* have not been widely used in relation to pediatric patients and their families, there is plenty of evidence of persisting distress in a significant minority of both children and their parents following PICU treatment.[6-14]

In another recent review relevant to the care of pediatric patients,[15] a useful model is proposed to inform future research into PICS. This model distinguishes between "modifiable" and "non-modifiable" risk factors associated with the likelihood of developing PICS prior to ICU admission, during admission, and following discharge. The authors highlight the variability in studies to date, in relation to the tools used for measuring distress and the length and timing of follow-up, and call for more uniformity in relation to epidemiology so that we can develop appropriate evidence-based services for this vulnerable population.

Models of care in pediatrics have traditionally been more family-focused than those in adult settings. Meert et al.[16] have recently shown how the ethos of patient- and family-centered care (PFCC)[17] is currently being operationalized in PICUs. Four examples are provided in this review, all of which relate to the acute phase while the child is still receiving critical care treatment. These address (a) the development of family visiting policies; (b) the involvement of families in medical rounds; (c) encouragement of the presence of family members during resuscitation; and (d) the practice of holding regular family conferences to discuss treatment progress and aid in decision-making.

However, in order to inform our thinking about direct support for the child and to extend our attention to beyond the PICU—to aim for care "without walls"[18]—it is necessary to look to the subspecialty of pediatric psychology for inspiration. The generic Pediatric Medical Traumatic Stress (PMTS) model[19] was originally developed to guide treatment and research with the families of children with cancer, but it lends itself particularly well to the PICU setting, with its stress on potentially traumatizing events (PTEs) and its firm focus on the family. Appropriately, it also emphasizes how well the majority of families fare in the longer term, arguing that while interventions should be trauma-focused they should also be "brief, competency-based, and non-stigmatising." In relation to this focus on positive aspects, it is interesting to note that many PICU patients' parents report posttraumatic *growth* as well as posttraumatic stress.[20]

The PMTS model describes families' experience in three phases. In phase 1, "peri-trauma," an important goal of intervention is to change the subjective experience of PTEs, which are often recurrent in medical settings, by providing normative information about how people usually react—in order to help families anticipate how they and the patient are likely to feel in the short term. (There are parallels here with Davidson's suggestion that staff can help families in adult ICU settings with "sense-making"[21] and with the apparent value of involving psychologists early on in the care of adult ICU patients after traumatic injury.[22])

In phase 2, "evolving, ongoing treatment," when the child is still actively in treatment but may no longer be critically ill, the focus is still on preventative strategies with the aim of minimizing distress by mobilizing family coping and being alert to developmental considerations in the child. Then, in phase 3, "long term," the focus shifts to one of monitoring and treatment of persistent symptoms.

SUPPORT IN THE ACUTE PHASE

In the acute stage of medical treatment in the PICU, the emphasis, from a psychological perspective, is primarily preventative and initially focused on parental reactions at a time when the child is usually too unwell or sedated to communicate with directly. It is important to acknowledge parents' long established needs for hope, proximity, and clear information[23] in the early days of a PICU admission, when parents are bombarded by many distressing sights and sounds, both in relation to their own child's treatment and the experiences of other families around them. They may well benefit from some normative information on the usual range of parental reactions in this difficult situation.

There are, however, a number of misapprehensions regarding the features of this experience that make it so difficult. There is an assumption that the high-tech environment is particularly distressing for parents—and indeed, many former patients later report how sounds that remind them of the suction machine or the ventilator alarm trigger painful memories. However, research using the Parental Stressor Scale: PICU (PSS:PICU),[24] to examine the degree to which parents find different aspects of the PICU experience difficult, has shown that it is the impact on their role as parents that is the greatest source of stress.[25] Parents instinctively want to comfort their child but may be unable to hold them or communicate with them for many days. Their only option is to wait things out and trust a team of people they often have never met before with the one thing most precious to them—their child's life.

Another assumption often made by staff is that the sicker the child, the greater the parents' distress, but research has repeatedly shown that the relationship between the severity of the child's medical condition and parental distress is not a linear one.[6] The primary mediating factor seems to be the parent's *subjective perception* of how sick the child is, with one study showing that the parents reporting the highest levels of distress at follow-up were those who thought their child could have died.[9] This is an example of an early appraisal that can be worked with, in keeping with the emphasis in the PMTS model of intervening in the early stages to uncover and clarify parents' beliefs. It is also important to be aware of other issues that may be contributing to parents' distress acutely. These include witnessing distressing scenes on the unit (e.g., emergency resuscitation of another child) and being concerned about other children at home. In relation to siblings, parents are often grateful for advice on what to tell them and whether to bring them in to the hospital to visit.

As the child's condition stabilizes, delirium is another important consideration. It may be helpful to warn families that their child may initially react in an uncharacteristic way after extubation, particularly if the child has been sedated for a long time. There is as yet no consensus on how best to assess delirium in children, although a number of promising tools have been developed.[26] However, in a finding that is consistent with research on adult ICU patients,[27,28] there is evidence that approximately one in three children experience strange hallucinatory or delusional experiences while critically ill, and that memory for these experiences is a risk factor for later posttraumatic stress symptoms.[29] The content of children's memories of psychotic experiences is very similar to that reported by delirious adults in intensive care settings, frequently including a heightened sense of threat, bizarre visions, and, in some cases, unpleasant tactile hallucinations akin to the feeling of being crawled over by large bugs. This unexpectedly fearful presentation, which usually only lasts a couple of days, can be especially distressing to a parent who may be longing to speak to a child who has been unconscious for days but who pulls away from the parent, fearing that the parent is a source of danger rather than comfort. Education that this type of reaction is a possibility and is more likely the longer the child has been sedated[29] can be reassuring and increases the chance of a parent maintaining his or her own emotional equilibrium throughout this transition.

The child's own emotional reactions and understanding of the situation he or she awakens to now need to be addressed. If children remember little of the circumstances that led to their admission, they will be bewildered to find themselves in a place they do not recognize, connected to all sorts of strange machines. This "memory gap"[30] may mean they are spared recall of the more traumatic events that can later haunt their parents, but some children are disturbed, just as adult patients are, to find they have no knowledge of what has been happening. Child life specialists, play therapists, and pediatric psychologists have particular skills in communicating with children in this sort of setting and may enable the team caring for the children to get a better understanding of the child's concerns. These concerns are not always obvious and are not necessarily the same as those of their parents, whose experience of the PICU may be very different.

The developmental level of the child may actually be protective in some cases, as children's understanding of the world may preclude them from even considering the possibility that they could have died, whereas a parent may find this hard to forget for months. The child, in contrast, having no memory of being operated on or ventilated, may be very upset at finding he or she has been put in diapers or at the prospect of a relatively minor medical procedure on the ward. Parents, overwhelmed by the gravity of the situation and the complexities of medical terminology, often appreciate help finding developmentally appropriate words to use with the sick child (see Box 7.1 for some examples of explanations of delirium-related experiences for children of different ages).

Another approach with children who have had particularly traumatic or protracted admissions to the PICU is to provide a more detailed,

---

Box7.1   EXAMPLES OF AGE-APPROPRIATE EXPLANATIONS OF DELIRIUM-RELATED EXPERIENCES FOR CHILDREN

"Did you see scary things? That sometimes happens when you are very sick." (for a 4-year-old child)

"Have you been seeing/hearing/feeling weird or scary things while you were in the PICU? Other children have said that has happened to them. We think it sometimes happens because of all the medicines you have needed, but it usually goes away in a couple of days, and it doesn't mean you are going crazy." (for a 10-year-old child)

---

tangible explanation of events in the form of an individually tailored, age-appropriate storybook for the child,[26,31] as illustrated in Box 7.2, Case Study 1: Sophie, and in Figure 7.1. Although this approach has not yet been formally evaluated, it shares some commonalities with the COPE program,[32,33] an established intervention involving the provision of advice to parents and a generic storybook at hospital discharge that is associated with improved mental health outcomes in mothers and children a year after PICU treatment. There are also obvious comparisons here with adult ICU diaries, which are prepared in this acute phase and have also been found to be associated with lower rates of long-term psychopathology in adult critical illness survivors.[34-36]

Two subgroups of families deserve special mention here, families of regular patients in the PICU and those whose children die. Children on long-term ventilation may have long and recurrent stays in the PICU and, unlike the majority of children on these units, may be much more alert and aware of what is going on around them. At the same time they may have difficulty expressing their concerns because of their dependence on the ventilator. Noyes, who has studied this group of children and sought their views about their acute care, makes several useful recommendations for meeting their psychological needs.[37] Long-term PICU patients' parents, "frequent fliers" who are regularly on the unit because of their children's chronic conditions, are also a group worthy of special consideration. They report different needs and concerns from those of most

Box 7.2 CASE STUDY 1: SOPHIE, A 6-YEAR-OLD CHILD INVOLVED IN A CAR ACCIDENT, AND HER FATHER, MARK

Sophie, a 6-year-old girl, was traveling in the back seat of the family car on a trip to the airport for the family's annual vacation when the car was hit from the side by a small van. She sustained a serious fracture to her femur and briefly lost consciousness. In the crash, her mother, who was driving and seated on the same side of the car, sustained a serious head injury; but her father, although shocked, only sustained soft tissue injuries. Her baby sister, who was strapped into the seat next to her, was unhurt. Sophie's mother was airlifted to a hospital, as she was the most seriously injured, and Sophie traveled there in an ambulance soon afterward. Her father, who was trapped in the car, waited for emergency services to cut him and the baby free.

Sophie was sent for a CT scan on arrival at the hospital, as there was evidence that she had sustained an injury to the head, but thankfully the scan was unremarkable. She was, however, very distressed and confused and did not understand why her parents were not with her. She had no memory of the accident and had never visited the hospital before, as it was some distance from her home. By the time she was transferred from the operating room to the PICU, her father had been brought up to be with her, and he was by her bedside the following morning when she was extubated following surgery on her leg. The family was referred to the unit psychologist in view of Sophie's anxiety and the high level of distress in her father, who felt guilty that he had not been able to accompany Sophie to the hospital and was also worried about his wife, who was still unconscious in the adult ICU.

The intervention consisted of two parts: in the first week the focus was on promoting Mark's coping resources; subsequently, the psychologist's main goal was to aid Sophie's understanding of what had happened and to facilitate communication within the family. The psychologist met with Mark twice individually to help him think through his priorities with regard to a) getting adequate rest himself, b) keeping abreast of medical developments with his daughter and wife, and c) making arrangements for the care of the baby. The psychologist also obtained a detailed history of the main events of the accident in order to give a clear explanation to Sophie once she was sufficiently alert, as Mark was too upset and overwhelmed initially to do this without becoming very distressed. The psychologist used small toy figures to explain the sequence of events to Sophie and later made up an age-appropriate picture book for her to keep, once she was well enough to be transferred to the general ward. Sophie was relieved to hear that her mother was being cared for in the same hospital and that her grandmother was taking care of the baby. She was also pleased to discover that the police had arrested the van driver for dangerous driving. She was able to articulate that she had been very frightened upon first waking alone in the ambulance but now had a better understanding of why she had been brought to the hospital without her parents.

Two months later, in a follow-up telephone call, Sophie's parents reported that, after an initial period of clinginess, her behavior had largely returned to normal. When she returned to school, she brought the picture book to explain what had happened to her classmates and her teacher (Figure 7.1).

Mark, however, was still regularly experiencing flashbacks, particularly when he first tried to go to sleep at night. It was therefore suggested that, in order to monitor his symptoms of posttraumatic stress, anxiety, and depression, he should complete two sets of questionnaires 3 months apart, with a view to facilitating a local referral to mental health services if his symptoms persisted.

parents of children in the PICU for less than a week. Specifically, they express concerns about the quality of communication across the many services involved in the care of their child, and they do not always feel that their own extensive knowledge of their child's condition is appropriately acknowledged by the team caring for their child acutely.[38]

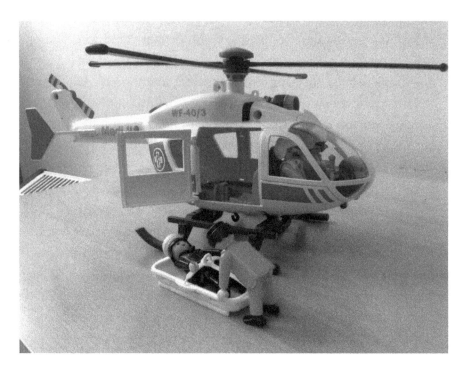

Figure 7.1. An illustration from a storybook made to help Sophie understand more about the events leading up to her intensive care admission.

Finally, the acute needs of parents who lose a child on the PICU have been sensitively examined in a number of qualitative studies, including one by Meyer and colleagues,[39] who found that parents appreciated honesty and a respect for the parent–child relationship, and another by Macdonald and colleagues,[40] who found that parents were particularly grateful for staff's small acts of kindness at the time of the child's death and their subsequent attendance at memorial services.

LONGER-TERM SUPPORT

The importance of speaking to children *directly* about their adjustment after difficult experiences is underlined by research in the fields of child psychology and pediatrics, which has shown that parents do not always fully appreciate their child's perspective. Depending on their own symptoms of posttraumatic stress, they are liable both to under- and overestimate how much their children are affected by traumatic events.[41] Despite being able to report accurately on their children's physical functioning, parents often report inaccurately on their children's emotional quality of life.[42] Notwithstanding these provisos, parents report that, for the most part, children, and especially very young children, recover well from an emotional/behavioral point of view after a PICU admission, although they may be wary of other adults for a time. However, parents also say that they are aware of a change in their parental relationship, in that they describe themselves as more fearful for their children, acknowledging that this can lead to overprotectiveness.[43]

Based on a series of qualitative interviews with children over 5 years of age and their parents, Atkins and colleagues[44] describe the overriding drive to return to "normal" that characterizes families' descriptions of the year following PICU discharge. For some, the definition of "normal" has to take account of markedly changed circumstances, such as a new diagnosis or uncertainty about prognosis, and for older children there is often a need to reassert their independence after a period of being unusually dependent on their parents. Another theme that emerges is the need to prioritize supporting the child's physical recovery before addressing what has happened, leading the authors to propose that a biopsychosocial framework is useful.

Even if a child is not reporting clinical levels of psychopathology, there may be a need, particularly in the case of chronic illness, for explanations regarding the critical phase to be updated regularly, to take account of the child's developing cognitive abilities. It will also sometimes be necessary to relate current treatment episodes to previous ones (see Box 7.3).

As noted, there is now considerable evidence that a significant minority of parents and children report elevated levels of distress—and particularly posttraumatic stress—after intensive care treatment, just as adult patients and their relatives do. Although most prevalence studies in this field are cross-sectional, there are also a number of prospective studies[45–47] which indicate that these symptoms persist for many months after discharge (see

---

Box 7.3   EXAMPLES OF AGE-APPROPRIATE EXPLANATIONS OF A RECURRING MEDICAL PROBLEM

"The doctor took away a lump in your tummy that was hurting." (for a 3-year-old child)

"You had a tumor in your tummy when you were 3 years old. The doctors took it out, but it has grown back, so they are going to take it out again and give you some medicine to try to stop it from coming back." (for an 8-year-old child with a recurrence of an earlier condition)

---

also Figure 7.2), leading the author of a recent editorial to argue that we now have a moral obligation to provide ongoing support for PICU families, not just during admission but after discharge, too.[48] Sadly, in practice, given that it is currently unusual for units to follow up with patients or families from a psychological perspective, it may be some time before their distress comes to the attention of an appropriate service.

As is the case in the parallel literature on adult ICU survivors,[15] we still understand relatively little about the risk factors for poor psychological

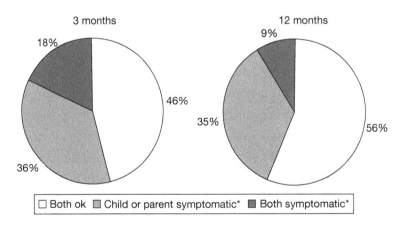

Figure 7.2. Proportions of child–parent pairs ($n = 66$) reporting clinically significant levels of posttraumatic stress symptoms at 3 and 12 months after discharge from a PICU (adapted from Colville and Pierce, 2012,[45] with permission).

outcomes in PICU patients and their families. Ward-Begnoche[49] points out that there are a number of potentially traumatizing aspects of this situation, relating both to the child's injuries or medical problems and to the treatment for their conditions. There does, however, seem to be an independent association between memories of frightening psychotic experiences and posttraumatic stress symptoms,[29] just as has been found with adults, which suggests that when presented with a clearly symptomatic child after PICU discharge, health professionals would do well to inquire about any particularly unusual experiences, dreams, or hallucinations they may have had during admission.

One promising tool to screen parents for risk of later distress is the Posttraumatic Adjustment Scale (PAS).[50] Although developed with an adult injury sample, it has been shown in a recent pilot study to be a useful tool to identify parents at risk of significant distress after their child's PICU admission.[51] Other examples of standardized measures that have be used to screen parents after their child's PICU stay are the Parental Stressor Scale: Pediatric Intensive Care Unit (PSS:PICU),[24] which predicts later parental distress[52] and those most likely to benefit from a follow-up clinic intervention;[53] the Acute Stress Disorder Scale (ASDS),[54] which was used prospectively in another study[9]; and a measure developed for use in the emergency room, the Screening Tool for Early Predictors of PTSD (STEPP),[55] which predicts posttraumatic stress symptoms in children and parents after injury.

Also, in relation to designing responsive services in the future, although we do not have a great deal of information on symptom trajectories in this group, it is important to consider the possibility of delayed reactions, which were found in nearly half of parents and children who were symptomatic at 1 year, in the study by Colville and Pierce.[45] These findings are consistent with the wider literature on posttraumatic stress disorder (PTSD), in which there is a growing appreciation of the extent to which symptoms may fluctuate over time. Bryant and colleagues[56] followed up a large sample of adult injury victims at several different points over a 2-year period and found that while most participants' symptoms remained in the nonclinical range, there were many examples of individuals who switched categorical status between "nonsymptomatic," "borderline," and "clinically significant" over time. It is unclear why some people later reported higher levels of symptoms, but the authors of this study did find associations with adverse life experiences in the intervening time period and with mild traumatic brain injury. These findings clearly have implications for the screening and monitoring of patients and families after intensive care treatment, since they suggest that one-time screening in the immediate aftermath of an admission could falsely eliminate many of those with debilitating symptoms at 1 year.

These results are also consistent with an important assumption of the PMTS model, namely that it is important not to ignore subsyndromal presentations referred to as *PTSS*—that is, posttraumatic stress *symptoms* which do not meet criteria for PTSD. Clinical experience over the years at our center, where there is dedicated pediatric psychology provision for the PICU and beyond, has shown that families appreciate being able to come back to the hospital where their child was treated and to dip in and out of treatment, as needed. We have noticed that levels of PTSS in different family members fluctuate and are exacerbated by sudden deteriorations in the child, particularly if this results in readmission to the hospital, which in turn brings repeated exposure to trauma triggers associated with the original admission.

For parents with frank and persisting symptoms of posttraumatic stress, there are a number of evidence-based treatments available.[57] One example of a brief treatment package is narrative exposure therapy,[58] the use of which is illustrated in Box 7.4, Case Study 2: Jane, and Figure 7.3, in which it became clear that, for this mother, the PICU admission was a stark reminder of her previously unresolved experiences on a neonatal unit. This treatment was originally devised for use with populations affected by repeated traumatic events in the context of war and natural disaster,[59] but it seems to fit well with the way parents describe what has happened to them in terms of an onslaught of distressing experiences, with no time to process what is going on emotionally, as opposed to a single-incident trauma.

Box 7.4 CASE STUDY 2: JANE, MOTHER OF STEVIE, AN 18-MONTH-OLD CHILD ADMITTED WITH CROUP

Jane, the mother of an 18-month-old child, Stevie, who was admitted to the PICU with croup, was referred acutely for support. It transpired that her son had been hospitalized for 6 months following his premature birth at 29 weeks and had had several apneic attacks during his stay on the neonatal unit. She had been very anxious at that time and had found it helpful to speak to the neonatal counselor then. However, although she thought that she had managed to put events behind her, she was reminded of them again during the present admission. Her son developed parainfluenza A and had a stormy course on the PICU which involved two failed extubations. Significantly, in terms of the impact on her mental health, another child of a similar age and with a similar medical history died after a sudden respiratory arrest in the bed next to her son, just before he was due to be discharged.

The psychologist met with the mother on three occasions while the child was still an inpatient, initially on the PICU and then twice on the general ward, and the psychologist offered to see the mother again following discharge if she found that her distress persisted.

Three months later, the respiratory pediatrician who was responsible for the child's medical follow-up requested that the psychologist see Jane again since, although Stevie had made a good recovery, his mother had become very tearful during a recent outpatient appointment, saying she felt unable to leave Stevie, who was sleeping in her bedroom, with anyone else.

The pediatric psychologist who had met Jane during Stevie's PICU admission screened her for symptoms and found that she was scoring above clinical cut-offs for anxiety and posttraumatic stress but not for depression. Further clinical interviewing established that she met full criteria for a diagnosis of posttraumatic stress disorder (PTSD) in relation to her experiences on the PICU. The psychologist therefore offered Jane a brief eight-session bi-weekly evidence-based treatment for this condition, narrative exposure therapy.[58] This involved Jane going over in detail what had happened and, with the therapist's help, constructing a written account of her life to date, incorporating the traumatic events on the PICU and on the neonatal unit. As part of this work, Jane was also encouraged to draw up a timeline of events, indicating particular highs and lows. With this whole life perspective, she was then asked to reflect on the thoughts and feelings the traumatic admission had brought up for her and to think about what she hoped for in the future.

Jane's symptoms were monitored at regular intervals over the following year. Three months after treatment her symptoms were significantly improved, in that she no longer met criteria for PTSD. Six months after treatment she felt able to return Stevie to his own bedroom, and she was discharged at 1 year, given that the improvement in her symptoms was maintained. She explained she had never felt before that she had been able to tell the whole story of her difficult experiences in the hospital, and she was now more able to get a sense of perspective on all that had happened. She said that she felt a burden had been lifted and that she was now able to get on with life and enjoy her child. Stevie continued to be monitored regularly but did not require further hospital admission.

Although the PTSD treatment literature on adults is much larger, there is also evidence that trauma-focused cognitive-behavioral therapy is also effective with children.[60] A recent case report in the pediatric literature shows how this approach has been successfully used with a PICU survivor.[61]

Finally, in relation to the special situation of bereavement in the PICU, Meert and colleagues have noted the particular risk of complicated grief reactions[62] and make useful recommendations for ways to structure contact with families after discharge in such a way that is most likely to be helpful.[63]

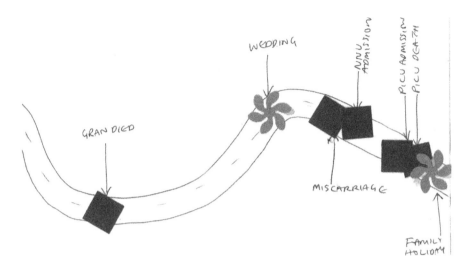

Figure 7.3. Jane's lifeline, drawn up as part of her treatment for PTSD using narrative exposure therapy. Some personal details have been changed to protect the patient's anonymity.

FUTURE DIRECTIONS

The recent priorities outlined by the latest SCCM task force charged with improving services to address PICS and PICS-F[64] are just as relevant to pediatric settings as they are to adult settings. We need to work together to increase public awareness of the emotional aftermath of intensive care admission; to clarify which staff should take on the responsibility for facilitating communication with families; and to do more research on risk factors, symptom trajectories, and interventions. In this way, we will be better able to reduce the distress of the "inseparable dyad"[4]—the patient and their family member—in the best interests of the whole family's long-term health and well-being.

Traditionally, there has not been a culture of following up with patients after PICU treatment. Conventionally, the clinical responsibility for their management has been devolved back to the appropriate pediatric specialist or the primary care provider. However, the growing evidence of physical and cognitive, as well as psychological, morbidities related to critical care conditions and their treatment[65-69] suggests that there is a need for PICU teams to reconsider the extent of their clinical responsibility to their patients—in short, as has been argued elsewhere,[70] there is now a need for a "paradigm shift." Even if intensivists are not best equipped to treat their surviving patients' post-discharge complications, a strong argument can be made that they are the people best placed to monitor their patients for conditions they are known to be at risk of developing; to set up clear referral pathways to appropriate services already in existence; and, ideally, to design in-house services that can provide greater continuity of care for PICU families in the future.

REFERENCES

1. Tan T, Brett SJ, Stokes T; Guideline Development Group. Rehabilitation after critical illness: summary of NICE guidance. *BMJ*. 2009;338:b822.
2. Desai SV, Law TJ, Needham DM. Long-term complications of critical care. *Crit Care Med*. 2011;39(2):371–379.
3. Davidson JE, Powers K, Hedayat KM, et al. Clinical practice guidelines for support of the family in the patient-centered intensive care unit: American College of Critical Care Medicine Task Force 2004–2005. *Crit Care Med*. 2007;35(2):605–622.
4. Davidson JE. Time for a formal assessment, treatment and referral structure for families of intensive care unit patients. *Crit Care Med*. 2012;40(5):1675–1676.
5. Davidson JE. The family experience with intensive care unit care: more than mere satisfaction. *Crit Care Med*. 2011;39(5):1207–1208.
6. Davydow DS, Richardson LP, Zatzick DF, Katon WJ. Psychiatric morbidity in pediatric critical illness survivors: a comprehensive review of the literature. *Arch Pediatr Adolesc Med*. 2010;164(4):377–385.
7. Colville G. The psychologic impact on children of admission to intensive care. *Pediatr Clin North Am*. 2008;55(3):605–616.
8. Rennick JE, Rashotte J. Psychological outcomes in children following pediatric intensive care unit hospitalization: a systematic review of the research. *J Child Health Care*. 2009;13(2):128–149.
9. Balluffi A. Kassam-Adams N, Kazak A, Tucker M, Dominguez T, Helfaer M. Traumatic stress in parents of children admitted to the pediatric intensive care unit. *Pediatr Crit Care Med*. 2004;5(6):547–553.
10. Bronner MB, Knoester H, Bos AP, Last BF, Grootenhuis MA. Posttraumatic stress disorder (PTSD) in children after paediatric intensive care treatment compared to children who survived a major fire disaster. *Child Adolesc Psychiatry Ment Health*. 2008;2(1):9.

11. Colville GA, Gracey D. Mothers' recollections of the paediatric intensive care unit: associations with psychopathology and views on follow up. *Intensive Crit Care Nurs.* 2006;22(1):49–55.

12. Nelson LP, Gold JI. Posttraumatic stress disorder in children and their parents following admission to the pediatric intensive care unit: a review. *Pediatr Crit Care Med.* 2012;13(3):338–347.

13. Rees G, Gledhill J, Garralda ME, Nadel S. Psychiatric outcome following paediatric intensive care unit (PICU) admission: a cohort study. *Intensive Care Med.* 2004;30(8):1607–1614.

14. Davidson JE, Jones C, Bienvenu OJ. Family response to critical illness: Postintensive care syndrome—family. *Crit Care Med.* 2012;40(2):618–624.

15. Long AC, Kross EK, Davydow DS, Curtis JR. Posttraumatic stress disorder among survivors of critical illness: creation of a conceptual model addressing identification, prevention, and management. *Intensive Care Med.* 2014;40:820–829.

16. Meert KL, Clark J, Eggly S. Family-centered care in the pediatric intensive care unit. *Pediatr Clin North Am.* 2013;60(3):761–772.

17. Committee on Hospital Care and Institute for Patient- and Family-Centered Care. Patient- and family-centered care and the pediatrician's role. *Pediatrics.* 2012;129(2):394–404.

18. Hillman K. Critical care without walls. *Curr Opin Crit Care.* 2002;8(6):594–599.

19. Kazak AE, Kassam-Adams N, Schneider S, Zelikovsky N, Alderfer MA, Rourke M. An integrative model of pediatric medical traumatic stress. *J Pediatr Psychol.* 2006;31:343–355.

20. Colville G, Cream P. Post-traumatic growth in parents after a child's admission to intensive care: maybe Nietzsche was right? *Intensive Care Med.* 2009;35(5):919–923.

21. Davidson JE. Facilitated sensemaking: a strategy and new middle-range theory to support families of intensive care unit patients. *Crit Care Nurse.* 2010;30(6):28–39.

22. Peris A, Bonizzoli M, Iozzelli D et al. Early intra-intensive care unit psychological intervention promotes recovery from post-traumatic stress disorders, anxiety and depression symptoms in critically ill patients. *Crit Care.* 2011;15(1):R1.

23. Molter NC. Needs of relatives of critically ill patients: a descriptive study. *Heart Lung.* 1979;8(2):332–339.

24. Carter MC, Miles MS. The Parental Stressor Scale: pediatric intensive care unit. *Matern Child Nurs J.* 1989;18(3):187–198.

25. Curley MA, Wallace J. Effects of the nursing Mutual Participation Model of Care on parental stress in the pediatric intensive care unit—a replication. *J Pediatr Nurs.* 1992;7(6):377–385.

26. Colville G. Psychological aspects of the care of the critically ill child. *J Pediatr Intensive Care.* 2015;4(4):182–187.

27. Svenningsen H. Associations between sedation, delirium and post-traumatic stress disorder and their impact on quality of life and memories following discharge from an intensive care unit. *Dan Med J.* 2013;60(4):B4630.

28. Jones C, Griffiths RD, Humphris G, Skirrow PM. Memory, delusions and the development of acute posttraumatic stress disorder–related symptoms after intensive care. *Crit Care Med.* 2001;29(3):573–580.

29. Colville G, Kerry S, Pierce C. Children's factual and delusional memories of intensive care. Am J Respir Crit Care Med. 2008;177(9):976–982.
30. Griffiths RD, Jones C. Filling the intensive care memory gap? *Intensive Care Med.* 2001;27(2):344–346.
31. Colville G. Paediatric intensive care. *Psychologist.* 2012;25(3):206–209.
32. Melnyk BM, Alpert-Gillis L, Feinstein NF, et al. Creating opportunities for parent empowerment: program effects on the mental health/coping outcomes of critically ill young children and their mothers. *Pediatrics.* 2004;113(6):597–607.
33. Melnyk BM, Crean HF, Feinstein NF, Fairbanks E, Alpert-Gillis LJ. Testing the theoretical framework of the COPE program for mothers of critically ill children: an integrative model of young children's posthospital adjustment behaviors. *J Pediatr Psychol.* 2007;32(4):463–474.
34. Jones C, Bäckman C, Capuzzo M, et al; RACHEL Group. Intensive care diaries reduce new onset post-traumatic stress disorder following critical illness: a randomised, controlled trial. *Crit Care.* 2010;14(5):R168.
35. Knowles RE, Tarrier N. Evaluation of the effect of prospective patient diaries on emotional well-being in intensive care unit survivors: a randomized controlled trial. *Crit Care Med.* 2009;37(1):184–191.
36. Garrouste-Orgeas M, Coquet I, Perier A, et al. Impact of an intensive care unit diary on psychological distress in patients and relatives. *Crit Care Med.* 2012;40(7):2033–2040.
37. Noyes J. "Ventilator-dependent" children who spend prolonged periods of time in intensive care units when they no longer have a medical need or want to be there. *J Clin Nurs.* 2000;9(5):774–783.
38. Graham RJ, Pemstein DM, Curley MA. Experiencing the pediatric intensive care unit: perspective from parents of children with severe antecedent disabilities. *Crit Care Med.* 2009;37(6):2064–2070.
39. Meyer EC, Ritholz MD, Burns JP, Truog RD. Improving the quality of end-of-life care in the pediatric intensive care unit: parents' priorities and recommendations. *Pediatrics.* 2006;117(3):649–657.
40. Macdonald ME, Liben S, Carnevale FA, et al. Parental perspectives on hospital staff members' acts of kindness and commemoration after a child's death. *Pediatrics.* 2005;116(4):884–890.
41. Kassam-Adams N, Garcia-Espana JF, Miller VA, Winston F. Parent–child agreement regarding children's acute stress: the role of parent acute stress reactions. *J Am Acad Child Adolesc Psychiatry.* 2006;45(12):1485–1493.
42. Upton P, Lawford J, Eiser C. Parent–child agreement across child health-related quality of life instruments: a review of the literature. *Qual Life Res.* 2008;17:895–913.
43. Colville G, Darkins J, Hesketh J, Bennett V, Alcock J, Noyes J. The impact on parents of a child's admission to intensive care: integration of qualitative findings from a cross-sectional study. *Intensive Crit Care Nurs.* 2009;25(2):72–79.
44. Atkins E, Colville G, John M. A "biopsychosocial" model for recovery: a grounded theory study of families' journeys after a paediatric intensive care admission. *Intensive Crit Care Nurs.* 2012;28(3):133–140.

45. Colville G, Pierce C. Patterns of post-traumatic stress symptoms in families after paediatric intensive care. *Intensive Care Med.* 2012;38:1523–1531.

46. Le Brocque RM, Hendrikz J, Kenardy JA. The course of posttraumatic stress in children: examination of recovery trajectories following traumatic injury. *J Pediatr Psychol.* 2010;35(6):637–645.

47. Bronner MB, Peek N, Knoester H, Bos AP, Last BF, Grootenhuis MA. Course and predictors of posttraumatic stress disorder in parents after pediatric intensive care treatment of their child. *J Pediatr Psychol.* 2010;35(9):966–974.

48. Hoehn KS. Posttraumatic stress and technology: do extracorporeal membrane oxygenation programs have an ethical obligation to provide ongoing support for parents? *Pediatr Crit Care Med.* 2014;15:180–181.

49. Ward-Begnoche W. Posttraumatic stress symptoms in the pediatric intensive care unit. *J Spec Pediatr Nurs.* 2007;12(2):84–92.

50. O'Donnell ML, Creamer MC, Parslow R, et al. A predictive screening index for posttraumatic stress disorder and depression following traumatic injury. *J Consult Clin Psychol.* 2008;76(6):923–932.

51. Samuel V, Colville G, Goodwin S, Ryninks. Identifying parents at high risk of PTSD after their child's PICU admission: the value of a brief screening tool. *Pediatr Crit Care Med.* 2014;15(4):22.

52. Colville G, Cream P. Screening for post-traumatic stress in parents after their child's admission to PICU. *Pediatr Crit Care Med.* 2006;7(4):410.

53. Colville GA, Cream PR, Kerry SM. Do parents benefit from the offer of a follow-up appointment for their child's admission to intensive care?: an exploratory randomised controlled trial. *Intensive Crit Care Nurs.* 2010;26(3):146–153.

54. Bryant RA, Moulds MI, Guthrie RM. Acute Stress Disorder Scale: a self-report measure of acute stress disorder. *Psychol Assess.* 2000;12(1):61–68.

55. Ward-Begnoche WL, Aitken ME, Liggin R, et al. Emergency department screening for risk for post-traumatic stress disorder among injured children. *Inj Prev.* 2006;12(5):323–326.

56. Bryant RA, O'Donnell ML, Creamer M, McFarlane AC, Silove D. A multisite analysis of the fluctuating course of posttraumatic stress disorder. *JAMA Psychiatry.* 2013;70(8):840–846.

57. National Collaborating Centre for Mental Health (UK). *Post-Traumatic Stress Disorder: The Management of PTSD in Adults and Children in Primary and Secondary Care.* Leicester (UK): Gaskell; 2005.

58. Schauer M, Neuner F, Elbert T. *Narrative Exposure Therapy: A Short-Term Treatment for Traumatic Stress Disorders.* 2nd ed. Cambridge, MA: Hogrefe Publishing; 2011.

59. Robjant K, Fazel M. The emerging evidence for narrative exposure therapy: a review. *Clin Psychol Rev.* 2010;30(8):1030–1039.

60. Smith P, Perrin S, Dalgleish T, Meiser-Stedman R, Clark DM, Yule W. Treatment of posttraumatic stress disorder in children and adolescents. *Curr Opin Psychiatry.* 2013;26(1):66–72.

61. Bronner MB, Beer R, Jozine van Zelm van Eldik M, Grootenhuis MA, Last BF. Reducing acute stress in a 16-year old using trauma-focused cognitive behaviour

therapy and eye movement desensitization and reprocessing. *Dev Neurorehabil.* 2009;12(3):170–174.

62. Meert KL, Shear K, Newth CJ, et al; Eunice Kennedy Shriver National Institute of Child Health and Human Development Collaborative Pediatric Critical Care Research Network. Follow-up study of complicated grief among parents eighteen months after a child's death in the pediatric intensive care unit. *J Palliat Med.* 2011;14(2):207–214.

63. Eggly S, Meert KL, Berger J, et al; Eunice Kennedy Shriver National Institute of Child Health and Human Development Collaborative Pediatric Critical Care Research Network. A framework for conducting follow-up meetings with parents after a child's death in the pediatric intensive care unit. *Pediatr Crit Care Med.* 2011;12(2):147–152.

64. Elliott D, Davidson JE, Harvey MA, et al. Exploring the scope of post-intensive care syndrome therapy and care: engagement of non-critical care providers and survivors in a second stakeholders meeting. *Crit Care Med.* 2014;42(12):2519–2526.

65. Dominguez TE. Are we exchanging morbidity for mortality in pediatric intensive care? *Pediatr Crit Care Med.* 2014;15(9):898–899.

66. Morrison W. Surviving and thriving after intensive care. *Pediatr Crit Care Med.* 2013;14(2):233–234.

67. Colville GA, Pierce CM. Children's self-reported quality of life after intensive care treatment. *Pediatr Crit Care Med.* 2013;14(2):e85–92.

68. Als LC, Nadel S, Cooper M, Pierce CM, Sahakian BJ, Garralda ME. Neuropsychologic function three to six months following admission to the PICU with meningoencephalitis, sepsis, and other disorders: a prospective study of school-aged children. *Crit Care Med.* 2013;41(4):1094–1103.

69. Bronner MB, Knoester H, Sol JJ, Bos AP, Heymnand HS, Grootenhuis MA. An explorative study on quality of life and psychological and cognitive function in pediatric survivors of septic shock. *Pediatr Crit Care Med.* 2009;10(6):636–642.

70. Needham DM, Davidson J, Cohen H, et al. Improving long-term outcomes after discharge from intensive care unit: report from a stakeholders' conference. *Crit Care Med.* 2012;40(2):502–509.

8

Family Response to Critical Illness

JUDY E. DAVIDSON AND GIORA NETZER

INTRODUCTION

Families exposed to the stress of a loved one's critical illness may suffer from a variety of health disturbances. The current chapter explores what we know about the family response to critical illness, both family intensive care unit syndrome (FICUS) and post-intensive care unit-family (PICS-F), as well as proposed interventions to prevent, mitigate, or treat these negative outcomes. We review what is known about the incidence of these adverse outcomes, including studies centered on intensive care unit (ICU) patients of all ages. Causal relationships are not clear, and preventive and treatment interventions are largely theorized—not fully tested. Nevertheless, it is our ethical duty to evaluate and treat the family to the best of our current ability. According to the precautionary principle, it is professionally acceptable to take action in the best interest of the family despite uncertainty regarding the effect of the intervention.[1] Knowing that family members will need the strength and mental aptitude to help with caregiving duties after discharge,[2,3] we have an obligation to do everything possible to support them with efforts towards health maintenance. It is no longer acceptable to focus exclusively on the patient, without considering the effect of a critical illness on the family.[4,5]

FAMILY INTENSIVE CARE UNIT SYNDROME

An adverse reaction to a loved one's critical illness can begin during the loved one's intensive care unit (ICU) stay. These acute adverse family outcomes have been termed "family ICU syndrome" (FICUS).[6] The proposed factors that underlie FICUS are: maladaptive reasoning, cognitive bias, high-intensity emotions, sleep deprivation, personal and family conflict, and anticipatory grief.

The stress of the ICU experience may overwhelm the coping mechanisms of family members. They may develop "learned helplessness," becoming resigned to the thought that there is nothing they can do to improve the situation, with resulting stress, anxiety, depression, disengagement, or withdrawal. Over half of family members appear to suffer from learned helplessness in the ICU setting.[7] Though we advocate shared decision-making,[8] learned helplessness makes it difficult for families to participate in the decision-making process.[7]

Providing families with structured activities during their loved one's ICU stay may decrease feelings of helplessness and facilitate improved coping. One proposed preventive measure, termed Facilitated Sensemaking, is to teach families how to participate in bedside activities (e.g., passive range of motion exercises, coaching during mobility efforts, and reading to the patient). This approach includes encouraging and praising family engagement, as well as thanking family members for their contributions during rounds and family meetings. Through proactively communicating with the family as a partner in healing, the family may experience a sense of purpose that, regardless of the patient's outcome, may serve as a protective factor for family health.[9-11]

Family integrity is also threatened by new and unexpected shifts in roles. Family inclusion in care can help provide role clarification and preserve family integrity.[12,13] Families report that inclusion by nurses supports role clarification. Role clarification through inclusion and engagement in bedside activities promotes family integrity by fostering a sense of agency.[14,15] Results from a qualitative study of parents of neonatal ICU (NICU) patients suggest that being involved in activities such as kangaroo care (holding a baby with skin-to-skin contact) and breastfeeding provide role clarification and a sense of purpose.[15]

For families with premature infants, the Neonatal Individualized Developmental Care and Assessment Program (NIDCAP) provides a structured approach to help the infants mature. One component of the NIDCAP approach involves trained facilitators teaching families how to engage with their babies at the bedside, with the goals of increased bonding, kangaroo care, and breastfeeding. Child outcomes from NIDCAP trials are inconsistent.[16-19] In a small RCT, mothers provided NIDCAP reported a significantly greater feeling of attachment to their babies; however, they also reported greater anxiety (which may simply reflect increased bonding).[19] In a comprehensive review of research conducted to explore the family response to pediatric critical illness, family coping improved with active participation in care.[20]

Family coping and confidence can also improve when communication is perceived as clear and complete.[20,21] Conversely, inadequate communication is a risk factor for clinician-family conflicts, prolonged ICU stays, increased hospital costs, and family members' developing post-traumatic stress disorder (PTSD).[22-25] Health care team members should be aware that gender issues may arise while promoting family engagement. In one qualitative study, fathers of NICU babies described that, in the hospital, the nurses were experts and assumed the primary caregiving responsibilities; following discharge, their wives took over this role, leaving them without a primary purpose. Returning to work to provide for the family helped fathers achieve a sense of purpose.[26] Given this, it seems prudent for nurses to consider creating special moments for fathers to promote attachment, bonding, and a sense of purpose and accomplishment while present with their babies or children. In the NICU, we advocate paternal kangaroo care. Gender stereotyping should be avoided (e.g., jumping to the conclusion that men would not be interested in direct care). Also, note that family members of ICU patients of all ages can participate in reading and storytelling to the patient, whether or not the family member feels comfortable with hands-on care.

Anger over the situation, fear of the unknown, and fear of patient death may be so intense that these feelings cloud a family member's thoughts and judgment. These high-intensity emotions may overwhelm a family member's ability to process environmental cues, and they can decrease his or her ability to participate meaningfully in the decision-making process. Anticipatory grief is similarly associated with impaired problem solving.[27] We propose that families whose cognitive processes are overwhelmed by emotion are prone to make emotion-based decisions that may not be aligned with the patient's values. Openly recognizing feelings of anger or fear during family conversations or meetings may help focus the distraught family.[6] We advocate structuring routine family meetings and allowing families to express their feelings prior to discussing changes in treatment plans.[28-30] At the patient's bedside, explaining equipment alarms and functions, as well as the importance or non-importance of sounds, may help reduce fear of the unknown.[9,10] Because families are in crisis, explanations may need to be repeated. Explaining why nurses may not respond immediately to each alarm has been shown to visibly decrease stress during observations of families at the bedside.[10]

Cognitive biases are common among family members of the critically ill. One of these is optimism bias, when a family has un-thwarted optimism despite warning signs of impending failure, or when a family holds out hope that a patient will be the 1 in a 100 who will survive an illness. In the ICU, families frequently misinterpret bad prognoses.[31,32] While this may allow the family to cope day-to-day, the ultimate result is a clouded perspective of reality, preempting adequate preparation for prolonged hospitalization, permanent disability, or death. On the other hand, families who engage in anticipatory grief may develop depression.[6] An acknowledgment addressing excessive optimism must be tempered with an understanding of the importance of hope among family members; hope is a potent protective factor.[33] Families validate that hope helps to deal with critical illness, even when prognosis is poor,[34,35] and it can be difficult to balance the duty to inform while fulfilling the family's need to preserve hope.[36]

Considering these barriers to clear thinking, we advocate the teach-back method of instruction to assure that information imparted is understood. This method includes providing information in small portions, and asking clarifying open-ended questions throughout the session to evaluate understanding.[37,38] If families understand the prognosis and potential outcomes, the clinician has fulfilled the duty to inform. Meeting information needs appears to help families cope,[34,39] and the need to maintain hope is important in the face of a poor prognosis.[34,35] Creating space in the dialogue not only for information, but also for hope, may be protective. As is common in palliative care practice, hope may be shifted with the goals of care; e.g. family members may hope for the ability to communicate together or for reduced patient pain. Articulating the word "hope" within these discussions may transparently communicate that the healthcare team understands the family's need.

Sleep deprivation is common in family members of the critically ill.[40-42] Over half of family members suffer excessive sleepiness, cognitive blunting from sleep deprivation, or both.[42] Since safeguarding is a natural instinct during crisis, during the acute phase of a critical illness, families may have a strong desire to stay overnight to be present for their sick loved one.[10,43,44] In order to encourage family presence at the bedside, newer ICU rooms are constructed with family space, including sleep areas,[8,45] but the lights, alarms, and routine ICU noise may also disrupt sleep. In units that do not have family sleep accommodations, sleep disruption is exacerbated when families sleep in bedside chairs or waiting room furniture not designed for sleep. For those families who sleep at home, anxiety related to separation combined with the unknown may prevent adequate rest, including sleep. Sleep disruption naturally results in physical fatigue and blunted cognitive functioning that may have negative effects on perceived stress and decision-making,[40,46,47] Families themselves suggest that sleep quality would improve if they were provided more information and taught relaxation techniques,[40] as anxiety reduces sleep quality.[48]

Because each family member copes with the situation in a unique manner, intra-family conflict may arise. Because this strain occurs during crisis, memories enhanced by strong negative feelings may persist well past hospitalization and threaten family integrity.[20,49,50] Family members may also be upset when they witness conflict within the healthcare team,[49] or when they feel that the healthcare team does not approve of how they are responding to the situation.[51,52] It is important to assess families for role strain and offer listening, advice, and referrals if indicated to social services, chaplains, or clinicians with mental health expertise.

POST–INTENSIVE CARE SYNDROME–FAMILY

Adverse family responses to a loved one's critical illness have been recognized by the Society of Critical Care Medicine as post–intensive care syndrome–family (PICS-F).[53] While FICUS is focused on family issues during the ICU stay, PICS-F begins in the ICU, may relate to the

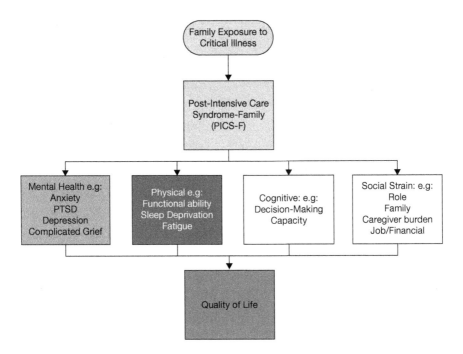

Figure 8.1. Post–intensive care syndrome in families (PICS-F).
Reprinted with permission from Davidson JE, McDuffie M, Campbell K. Family centered care. In: Goldsworthy S, Kleinpell RM, Speed G, eds. *Best Practices in Global Critical Care Nursing*. New York: Springer, 2017.

ICU events described, continues through transfer, and lingers follow-ing patient discharge or death. PICS-F originally included only mental health outcomes, but the first author (JD) has proposed an expansion to highlight physical and social problems as well (see Figure 8.1).[54] Resolution of these disturbances may take months to years; long-term studies are needed to track epidemiologic patterns of symptom resolu-tion. Most of what is known about PICS-F comes from studies lasting a year, at most.[55]

ANXIETY, POSTTRAUMATIC STRESS DISORDER, AND DEPRESSION

Symptoms of anxiety, PTSD, and depression occur in roughly 40% (13-56%), 21% (13-56%), and 23% (21-56%) of family members within the first several months after ICU discharge.[56-58] In addition, acute stress symptoms have been reported in a third of parents of critically ill chil-dren.[56,58] Demographic risk factors include being female or a single par-ent of a critically ill child. Though evidence regarding educational level as a risk factor is conflicting,[59,60] a prior history of anxiety, depression or other mental illness is also associated with a higher post-ICU burden of distress.[56,61-63] The patients' ICU length of stay does not appear to predict anxiety or depression in family members.[64]

Health care team behavior may impact long-term family psychological outcomes. Families report increased psychological disturbances when the physician was not perceived as comforting.[65] In a study of family mem-bers of patients who experienced out-of-hospital cardiac arrest, those who perceived that the patient's treatment was inadequate experienced higher rates of PTSD.[62]

From studies of family members of terminal cancer patients, we know that witnessing delirium in loved ones can cause substantial psychologi-cal distress, including feelings of helplessness, anxiety, and exhaustion. Therefore, we recommend providing delirium-specific support and infor-mation to families.[66] Early patient mobility is a known measure to prevent delirium in critically ill patients.[67] Teaching family members range-of-motion exercises and engaging them as mobility coaches could promote a sense of agency in delirium prevention and care giving.[68]

Acutely, families seek information to decrease anxiety and stress.[69] Their ability to receive this information may also have long-lasting effects. Family members who perceive communication as incomplete appear to have more post-discharge PTSD symptoms.[70] When structured communication is provided to help with shared decision-making during withdrawal of life support, anxiety and stress can be reduced.[71] In an observational study related to decision-making anxiety, stress was decreased when families perceived clear and consistent communication.[72] The VALUE method of case conferencing (value family contributions, acknowledge emotions, listen, understand the patient as a human, elicit questions from the family)[28,29] focuses on providing empathic statements and active listening. Structured family conferences coupled with a brochure were associated with decreased symptoms of anxiety (45 vs. 67%), post-traumatic stress (45 vs. 69%) and depression (29 vs. 56%).[73] In another study brochures alone did not decrease anxiety, however, increased staff-family interaction significantly improved anxiety. Authors concluded that limited staff communication was a key factor contributing to family anxiety.[74] Communication may also be enhanced through family participation in rounds. Parents have reported that involvement in NICU rounds decreases stress while improving confidence in the healthcare team.[75] Family participation in rounds is endorsed by the American College of Critical Care Medicine (ACCM)/Society of Critical Care Medicine (SCCM).[8]

Family presence at cardiopulmonary resuscitation is controversial and known to cause staff stress. However, when requested by the family the practice is endorsed by the ACCM/SCCM[8] and the American Association of Critical Care Nurses.[76] Interestingly, accepting an invitation to witness a family member's pre-hospital resuscitation attempts, if anything, appears protective against subsequent PTSD, anxiety, and depression.[77,78]

To reduce the risk of future distress—including PTSD—in patients and family members, a popular European communication strategy is ICU diaries. As noted in Chapter 6, these diaries are written to the patient by staff and, often, family members themselves. Caring, hope, concern, and information are conveyed in short daily entries. Nurses take care to explain noxious stimuli that are often misconstrued by patients and remembered. Even though the diaries are meant to help the patient reconstruct their illness narrative post-discharge, they have also been associated with decreased PTSD in family members.[79,80] Looking back to the discussion regarding facilitated sensemaking and family engagement at the bedside, writing diary entries may give family members a sense of purpose during crisis, minimize their sense of helplessness, and provide an opportunity for daily processing of in-ICU and outside events. There may be a benefit to the real time de-fragmentation of distorted perceptions of events, for both patients and family members.[81,82] The caring messages written by staff may also have a therapeutic effect on families.[83]

For mothers of infants in the NICU, peer-to-peer support is helpful for maternal role processing and breastfeeding skills.[84–86] Similar programs have not been studied in adult ICUs, but demonstration projects are in progress through the SCCM (http://www.sccm.org/Research/Quality/thrive/Pages/default.aspx, accessed 3/17/2016). Families can also be referred to disease-specific support groups (e.g., the Sepsis Alliance http://www.sepsisalliance.org or the ARDS Foundation www.ardsusa.org). The popularity of these groups is a testimony to their perceived benefit; however, research to support further development of peer-to-peer programs is sorely needed.

The transition out of the ICU may also impact family distress, which can be reduced by purposely providing information.[87,88] Family brochures explaining PICS-F are available through www.sccm.org. Feedback from families who learn about PICS-F to the first author (JD) indicates that it is helpful to know that they are not alone in their experiences.

COMPLICATED GRIEF

Complicated grief (prolonged, intense bereavement-related dysphoria) affects approximately 10% of bereaved family members and is more common in women.[63] Symptoms may include intense yearning for the deceased, preoccupation with thoughts about them, avoidance, anger, and disbelief.[63] As with other psychological distress phenomena, accepting an offer to witness resuscitation efforts is associated with reduced later grief.[78] Optimizing family communication with clinical staff and the patient appears beneficial, perhaps particularly for those family members who live alone.[63]

CAREGIVING BURDEN

More than half of the patients discharged from an ICU will require caregiving at home,[2,3] and caregiving can lead to emotional distress, relationship strain, and physical exhaustion.[89,90] The burden is higher when the caregiver is not prepared to assume this role and lower when family members have some degree of mastery and good social support.[89] Female sex is an independent risk factor for caregiver burden. Additional risk factors include hours of caregiving, depression, financial stress, and having no choice in being a caregiver.

The burden of caring for chronically critically ill children on ventilators at home can be overwhelming.[91] Families feel isolated not only due to their caregiving responsibilities but also due to the response they receive from others who question their choice to provide this treatment (as opposed to allowing their child to die).[91]

It is prudent to prepare family members early in a critical illness regarding the patient's likely need for caregiving afterward. Teaching family members simple caregiving tasks while their loved one is hospitalized can provide a sense of purpose during the acute phase of illness, as well as confidence after discharge. Family presence in the hospital allows family members to witness expert care delivery and facilitates mastery of skills they may be required to assume in the home.

PHYSICAL OUTCOMES

As discussed, inadequate sleep is common among family members of critically ill patients, especially early in the ICU admission. Sleeplessness, fatigue, and worsening general health are also common complications of caregiving and bereavement following discharge or death.[92,93] In one study of 47 family members of critical illness survivors, half reported clinically significant fatigue that was associated with depressive symptoms, greater health risk behaviors, poor sleep quality, and physical symptoms.[93] Importantly, fatigue is a predictive indicator of worsening disease and illness, increased use of healthcare resources, and shortened life expectancy.[93]

SOCIAL OUTCOMES

Role strain and Family Integrity

Long-term role strain, marital problems, and changes in relationships result from the burden of enduring critical illness and caregiving.[20,94-97] For example, in a study of parents of critically ill children who had been in the NICU, both mothers and fathers reported a significant ($p < 0.0001$) decrease in family function 1 year post-discharge.[98]

In neonates, family integrity is threatened by barriers to bonding in the NICU. Separation of parents while their babies are in the NICU may result in poorly-formed empathy for the child and neglect or abuse post-discharge. In one study, a NICU webcam was provided with the goal of increasing parental bonding with infants despite separation (due to work/financial obligations). The authors reported positive uptake of the webcam by parents and decreased anxiety during separation. Long-term outcomes have not yet been reported.[99] Medical technology and ICU interventions also prevent parents from bonding after high-risk births. With appropriate parental support and communication about the infant's status, however, nurses can facilitate attachment.[100]

Further research is needed to quantify the magnitude of these burdens and identify best-treatment options. Psychological or marital counseling may be needed long-term to cope with the continued burden of caregiving and to deal with the long-term aftermath of exposure to traumatic events in critical illness and intensive care.[56,101]

Return to Work and Financial Strain

Returning to work may be impractical or impossible due to caregiving responsibilities and/or psychological disturbances following a loved one's critical illness. Financial difficulties are incurred when family members cannot return to work, or if the cost of care exceeds the family's budget. However, as noted, fathers of babies in the NICU reported that returning to work gave them a sense of purpose given their marginalized role at the bedside. Providing for the family during and after the critical illness became a focal point of coping and comfort, though juggling work vs. caregiving responsibilities can be stressful.[26] Long-term hospitalizations can predictably create a financial burden for families, whether or not their loved ones survive. In a survey of family members of adult patients who had died in the ICU, nearly a third had financial difficulties, and less than half of those previously employed had returned to work when interviewed a median of 33 days after death.[92] Additional studies are needed of the financial implications of critical illnesses on families and society.

Quality of life

Quality of life of family members of critically ill patients is affected by lingering mental health concerns, as well as caregiving and financial burdens. Suggestions to improve quality of life include conflict prevention and resolution, psychiatric support during or following the ICU stay, and better end-of-life care.[55,102] Pilot clinics and post-ICU demonstration projects are being tested in the United States given the known problems of critical illness survivors and their family members. We are increasingly recognizing that we have an unmet need to create a specialty of mental health clinicians who can knowledgably treat persons exposed to critical illness and intensive care.

CONCLUSION

Family members of ICU patients can have mental, physical, and social responses to critical illness. These responses can begin when their loved ones are in the ICU and persist after discharge. Interventions in the ICU could have long-term effects on family members. Communication, proximity, engagement, maintaining family integrity, optimizing sleep, and conflict resolution may all play a role in family health following the discharge or death of the patient. Research is needed to further quantify the epidemiology, mechanisms of action, and efficacy of interventions to optimize the health of this large group of people. While waiting for research results to definitively point us towards effective preventive measures and early interventions, it is prudent to optimize communication, encourage proximity and engagement, and support the health of family members while caring for the critically ill and injured. As patients and their families move into the home environment, it is important to consider their long-term health as well.

REFERENCES

1. Upshur RE. Evidence and ethics in public health: the experience of SARS in Canada. *N S W Public Health Bull.* 2012;23(5-6):108–110.
2. Desai SV, Law TJ, Needham DM. Long-term complications of critical care. *Crit Care Med.* 2011;39(2):371–379.
3. Unroe M, Kahn JM, Carson SS, et al. One-year trajectories of care and resource utilization for recipients of prolonged mechanical ventilation: a cohort study. *Ann Intern Med.* 2010;153(3):167–175.
4. American Nurses Association. *Code of Ethics for Nurses with Interpretive Statements,* 2nd ed. Silver Spring, MD: Nursebooks.org; 2015, p. 76.

5. Davidson JE. Time for a formal assessment, treatment, and referral structure for families of intensive care unit patients. *Crit Care Med.* 2012;40(5):1675–1676.

6. Netzer G, Sullivan DR. Recognizing, naming, and measuring a family intensive care unit syndrome. *Ann Am Thorac Soc.* 2014;11(3):435–441.

7. Sullivan DR, Liu X, Corwin DS, et al. Learned helplessness among families and surrogate decision-makers of patients admitted to medical, surgical, and trauma ICUs. *Chest.* 2012;142(6):1440–1446.

8. Davidson JE, Powers K, Hedayat KM, et al. Clinical practice guidelines for support of the family in the patient-centered intensive care unit: American College of Critical Care Medicine Task Force 2004–2005. *Crit Care Med.* 2007;35(2):605–622.

9. Davidson JE. Facilitated sensemaking: a strategy and new middle-range theory to support families of intensive care unit patients. *Crit Care Nurse.* 2010;30(6):28–39.

10. Davidson JE, Daly BJ, Agan D, Brady NR, Higgins PA. Facilitated sensemaking: a feasibility study for the provision of a family support program in the intensive care unit. *Crit Care Nurs Q.* 2010;33(2):177–189.

11. Weick KE. *Sensemaking in Organizations.* Thousand Oaks, CA: Sage; 1995.

12. Tomlinson PS, Peden-McAlpine C, Sherman S. A family systems nursing intervention model for paediatric health crisis. *J Adv Nurs.* 2012;68(3):705–714.

13. Van Horn E, Tesh A. The effect of critical care hospitalization on family members: stress and responses. *Dimens Crit Care Nurs.* 2000;19(4):40–49.

14. Harbaugh BL, Tomlinson PS, Kirschbaum M. Parents' perceptions of nurses' caregiving behaviors in the pediatric intensive care unit. *Issues Compr Pediatr Nurs.* 2004;27(3):163–178.

15. Lasiuk GC, Comeau T, Newburn-Cook C. Unexpected: an interpretive description of parental traumas' associated with preterm birth. *BMC Pregnancy Childbirth.* 2013;13 Suppl 1:S13.

16. Als H, McAnulty GB. The Newborn Individualized Developmental Care and Assessment Program (NIDCAP) with kangaroo mother care (KMC): comprehensive care for preterm infants. *Curr Womens Health Rev.* 2011;7(3):288–301.

17. Ariagno RL, Thoman EB, Boeddiker MA, et al. Developmental care does not alter sleep and development of premature infants. *Pediatrics.* 1997;100(6):E9.

18. Blauw-Hospers CH, Hadders-Algra M. A systematic review of the effects of early intervention on motor development. *Dev Med Child Neurol.* 2005;47(6):421–432.

19. Kleberg A, Westrup B, Stjernqvist K, Lagercrantz H. Indications of improved cognitive development at one year of age among infants born very prematurely who received care based on the Newborn Individualized Developmental Care and Assessment Program (NIDCAP). *Early Hum Dev.* 2002;68(2):83–91.

20. Shudy M, de Almeida ML, Ly S, et al. Impact of pediatric critical illness and injury on families: a systematic literature review. *Pediatrics.* 2006;118(Suppl 3):S203–218.

21. Majesko A, Hong SY, Weissfeld L, White DB. Identifying family members who may struggle in the role of surrogate decision maker. *Crit Care Med.* 2012;40(8):2281–2286.

22. Breen CM, Abernethy AP, Abbott KH, Tulsky JA. Conflict associated with decisions to limit life-sustaining treatment in intensive care units. *J Gen Intern Med.* 2001;16(5):283–289.

23. Studdert DM, Mello MM, Burns JP, et al. Conflict in the care of patients with prolonged stay in the ICU: types, sources, and predictors. *Intensive Care Med.* 2003;29(9):1489–1497.

24. Teno JM, Fisher E, Hamel MB, et al. Decision-making and outcomes of prolonged ICU stays in seriously ill patients. *J Am Geriatr Soc.* 2000;48(5 Suppl): S70–74.

25. Siegel MD, Hayes E, Vanderwerker LC, Loseth DB, Prigerson HG. Psychiatric illness in the next of kin of patients who die in the intensive care unit. *Crit Care Med.* 2008;36(6):1722–1728.

26. Pohlman S. The primacy of work and fathering preterm infants: findings from an interpretive phenomenological study. *Adv Neonatal Care.* 2005;5(4):204–216.

27. Fowler NR, Hansen AS, Barnato AE, Garand L. Association between anticipatory grief and problem solving among family caregivers of persons with cognitive impairment. *J Aging Health.* 2013;25(3):493–509.

28. Curtis JR, Engelberg RA, Wenrich MD, et al. Studying communication about end-of-life care during the ICU family conference: development of a framework. *J Crit Care.* 2002;17(3):147–160.

29. Curtis JR, White DB. Practical guidance for evidence-based ICU family conferences. *Chest.* 2008;134(4):835–843.

30. Baile WF, Buckman R, Lenzi R, Glober G, Beale EA, Kudelka AP. SPIKES—A six-step protocol for delivering bad news: application to the patient with cancer. *Oncologist.* 2000;5(4):302–311.

31. Zier LS, Sottile PD, Hong SY, Weissfield LA, White DB. Surrogate decision makers' interpretation of prognostic information: a mixed-methods study. *Ann Intern Med.* 2012;156(5):360–366.

32. Lee Char SJ, Evans LR, Malvar GL, White DB. A randomized trial of two methods to disclose prognosis to surrogate decision makers in intensive care units. *Am J Respir Crit Care Med.* 2010;182(7):905–909.

33. Adams JA, Anderson RA, Docherty SL, Tulsky JA, Steinhauser KE, Bailey DE, Jr. Nursing strategies to support family members of ICU patients at high risk of dying. *Heart Lung.* 2014;43(5):406–415.

34. Chan KS, Twinn S. An analysis of the stressors and coping strategies of Chinese adults with a partner admitted to an intensive care unit in Hong Kong: an exploratory study. *J Clin Nurs.* 2007;16(1):185–193.

35. Engstrom A, Soderberg S. The experiences of partners of critically ill persons in an intensive care unit. *Intensive Crit Care Nurs.* 2004;20(5):299–308.

36. Apatira L, Boyd EA, Malvar G, et al. Hope, truth, and preparing for death: perspectives of surrogate decision makers. *Ann Intern Med.* 2008;149(12):861–868.

37. Fidyk L, Ventura K, Green K. Teaching nurses how to teach: strategies to enhance the quality of patient education. *J Nurses Prof Dev.* 2014;30(5):248–253.

38. Always use teach-back! Institute for Healthcare Improvement. http://www.ihi.org/resources/Pages/Tools/AlwaysUseTeachBack!.aspx. Accessed March 18, 2016.

39. Meyer EC, Ritholz MD, Burns JP, Truong RD. Improving the quality of end-of-life care in the pediatric intensive care unit: parents' priorities and recommendations. *Pediatrics.* 2006;117(3):649–657.

40. Day A, Haj-Bakri S, Lubchansky S, Mehta S. Sleep, anxiety and fatigue in family members of patients admitted to the intensive care unit: a questionnaire study. *Crit Care*. 2013;17(3):R91.
41. Van Horn E, Tesh A. The effect of critical care hospitalization on family members: stress and responses. *Dimens Crit Care Nurs*. 2000;19(4):40–49.
42. Verceles AC, Corwin DS, Afshar M, et al. Half of the family members of critically ill patients experience excessive daytime sleepiness. *Intensive Care Med*. 2014;40(8):1124–1131.
43. Burr G. Contextualizing critical care family needs through triangulation: an Australian study. *Intensive Crit Care Nurs*. 1998;14(4):161–169.
44. Davidson JE, Harvey MA, Schuller J, Black G. Post-intensive care syndrome: what to do and how to help prevent it. In *American Nurse Today*. American Nurses Association; 2013:32–38.
45. Thompson DR, Hamilton DK, Cadenhead CD, et al. Guidelines for intensive care unit design. *Crit Care Med*. 2012;40(5):1586–1600.
46. Kilgore W. Effects of sleep deprivation on cognition. In: Kerkhof G, Van Dongen H, eds. *Human Sleep and Cognition*. New York: Elsevier; 2010:105–131.
47. Busse M, Stromgren K, Thorngate L, Thomas KA. Parents' responses to stress in the neonatal intensive care unit. *Crit Care Nurse*. 2013;33(4):52–59.
48. Edéll-Gustafsson U, Angelhoff C, Johnsson E, Karlsson J, Mörelius E. Hindering and buffering factors for parental sleep in neonatal care. A phenomenographic study. *J Clin Nurs*. 2015;24(5-6):717–727.
49. Fassier T, Azoulay E. Conflicts and communication gaps in the intensive care unit. *Curr Opin Crit Care*. 2010;16(6):654–665.
50. Lutz K. Feeding problems of neonatal intensive care unit and pediatric intensive care unit graduates: perceptions of parents and providers. *Newborn Infant Nurs Rev*. 2012;12(4):207–213.
51. Soderstrom IM, Benzein E, Saveman BI. Nurses' experiences of interactions with family members in intensive care units. *Scand J Caring Sci*. 2003;17(2):185–192.
52. Hurst I. Vigilant watching over: mothers' actions to safeguard their premature babies in the newborn intensive care nursery. *J Perinat Neonatal Nurs*. 2001;15(3):39–57.
53. Needham DM, Davidson J, Cohen H, et al. Improving long-term outcomes after discharge from intensive care unit: report from a stakeholders' conference. *Crit Care Med*. 2012;40(2):502–509.
54. Davidson JE, McDuffie M, Campbell K. Family-centered care. In: Goldsworthy S, Kleinpell RM, Speed G, eds. *Best Practices in Global Critical Care Nursing*. New York: Springer; 2017.
55. Kentish-Barnes N, Lemiale V, Chaize M, Pochard F, Azoulay E. Assessing burden in families of critical care patients. *Crit Care Med*. 2009;37(10 Suppl):S448–456.
56. Davidson JE, Jones C, Bienvenu OJ. Family response to critical illness: post-intensive care syndrome-family. *Crit Care Med*. 2012;40(2):618–624.
57. Hartog CS, Schwarzkopf D, Riedemann NC, et al. End-of-life care in the intensive care unit: a patient-based questionnaire of intensive care unit staff perception and relatives' psychological response. *Palliat Med*. 2015;29(4):336–345.

58. Kong LP, Cui Y, Qiu YF, Han SP, Yu ZB, Guo XR. Anxiety and depression in parents of sick neonates: a hospital-based study. *J Clin Nurs*. 2013;22(7-8):1163–1172.

59. Kross EK, Engelberg RA, Gries CJ, Nielsen EL, Zatzick D, Curtis JR. ICU care associated with symptoms of depression and posttraumatic stress disorder among family members of patients who die in the ICU. *Chest*. 2011;139(4):795–801.

60. Kara S, Tan S, Aldemir S, Yilmaz A, Tatli M, Dilmen U. Investigation of perceived social support in mothers of infants hospitalized in neonatal intensive care unit. *Hippokratia*. 2013;17(2):130–135.

61. Plaszewska-Zywko L, Gazda D. Emotional reactions and needs of family members of ICU patients. *Anaesthesiol Intensive Ther*. 2012;44(3):145–149.

62. Zimmerli M, Tisljar K, Balestra GM, Langewitz W, Marsch S, Hunziker S. Prevalence and risk factors for post-traumatic stress disorder in relatives of out-of-hospital cardiac arrest patients. *Resuscitation*. 2014;85(6):801–808.

63. Kentish-Barnes N, Chaize M, Seegers V, et al. Complicated grief after death of a relative in the intensive care unit. *Eur Respir J*. 2015;45(5):1341–1352.

64. Hwang DY, Yagoda D, Perrey HM, et al. Anxiety and depression symptoms among families of adult intensive care unit survivors immediately following brief length of stay. *J Crit Care*. 2014;29(2):278–282.

65. Siegel MD, Hayes E, Vanderwerker LC, Loseth DB, Prigerson HG. Psychiatric illness in the next of kin of patients who die in the intensive care unit. *Crit Care Med*. 2008;36(6):1722–1728.

66. Partridge JS, Martin FC, Harari D, Dhesi JK. The delirium experience: what is the effect on patients, relatives and staff and what can be done to modify this? *Int J Geriatr Psychiatry*. 2013;28(8):804–812.

67. Barr J, Fraser GL, Puntillo K, et al. Clinical practice guidelines for the management of pain, agitation, and delirium in adult patients in the intensive care unit. *Crit Care Med*. 2013;41 (1):263–306.

68. Davidson JE, Harvey MA, Bemis-Dougherty A, Smith JM, Hopkins RO. Implementation of the pain, agitation, delirium clinical practice guidelines and promoting mobility to prevent post-intensive care syndrome. *Crit Care Med*. 2013;41(9 Suppl 1):S136–145.

69. Al-Mutair AS, Plummer V, Clerehan R, O'Brien A. Needs and experiences of intensive care patients' families: a Saudi qualitative study. *Nurs Crit Care*. 2014;19(3):135–144.

70. Azoulay E, Pochard F, Kentish-Barnes N, et al. Risk of post-traumatic stress symptoms in family members of intensive care unit patients. *Am J Respir Crit Care Med*. 2005;171(9):987–994.

71. Kryworuchko J, Hill E, Murray MA, Stacey D, Fergusson DA. Interventions for shared decision-making about life support in the intensive care unit: a systematic review. *Worldviews Evid Based Nurs*. 2013;10(1):3–16.

72. Iverson E, Celious A, Kennedy CR, et al. Factors affecting stress experienced by surrogate decision makers for critically ill patients: implications for nursing practice. *Intensive Crit Care Nurs*. 2014;30(2):77–85.

73. Lautrette A, Darmon M, Megarbane B, et al. A communication strategy and brochure for relatives of patients dying in the ICU. *N Engl J Med*. 2007;356(5):469–478.

74. Rusinova K, Kukal J, Simek J, Cerny V. Limited family members/staff communication in intensive care units in the Czech and Slovak Republics considerably increases anxiety in patients' relatives—the DEPRESS study. *BMC Psychiatry*. 2014;14:21.

75. Grzyb M, Coo H, Rühland L, Dow K. Views of parents and health-care providers regarding parental presence at bedside rounds in a neonatal intensive care unit. *J Perinatol*. 2014;34(2):143–148.

76. American Association of Critical-Care Nurses. Family presence during resuscitation and invasive procedures. http://www.aacn.org/wd/practice/content/family-presence-practice-alert.pcms?menu=practice. Accessed March 18, 2016.

77. Jabre P, Belpomme V, Azoulay E, et al. Family presence during cardiopulmonary resuscitation. *N Engl J Med*. 2013;368(11):1008–1018.

78. Jabre P, Tazarourte K, Azoulay E, et al. Offering the opportunity for family to be present during cardiopulmonary resuscitation: 1-year assessment. *Intensive Care Med*. 2014;40(7):981–987.

79. Garrouste-Orgeas M, Coquet I, Perier A, et al. Impact of an intensive care unit diary on psychological distress in patients and relatives. *Crit Care Med*. 2012;40(7):2033–2040.

80. Jones C, Backman C, Griffiths RD. Intensive care diaries and relatives' symptoms of posttraumatic stress disorder after critical illness: a pilot study. *Am J Crit Care*. 2012;21(3):172–176.

81. Backman CG, Walther SM. Use of a personal diary written on the ICU during critical illness. *Intensive Care Med*. 2001;27(2):426–429.

82. Egerod I, Christensen D, Schwartz-Nielsen KH, Ågård AS. Constructing the illness narrative: a grounded theory exploring patients' and relatives' use of intensive care diaries. *Crit Care Med*. 2011;39(8):1922–1928.

83. Gjengedal E, Storli SL, Holme AN, Eskerud RS. An act of caring: patient diaries in Norwegian intensive care units. *Nurs Crit Care*. 2010;15(4):176–184.

84. Rossman B, Greene MM, Meier PP. The role of peer support in the development of maternal identity for "NICU Moms". *J Obstet Gynecol Neonatal Nurs*. 2015;44(1):3–16.

85. Rossman B, Engstrom JL, Meier PP. Healthcare providers' perceptions of breast-feeding peer counselors in the neonatal intensive care unit. *Res Nurs Health*. 2012;35(5):460–474.

86. Levick J, Quinn M, Vennema C. NICU parent-to-parent partnerships: a comprehensive approach. *Neonatal Netw*. 2014;33(2):66–73.

87. Linton S, Grant C, Pellegrini J. Supporting families through discharge from PICU to the ward: the development and evaluation of a discharge information brochure for families. *Intensive Crit Care Nurs*. 2008;24(6):329–337.

88. Brooke J, Hasan N, Slark J, Sharma P. Efficacy of information interventions in reducing transfer anxiety from a critical care setting to a general ward: a systematic review and meta-analysis. *J Crit Care*. 2012;27(4):425.e429–415.

89. Cameron JI, Herridge MS, Tansey CM, McAndrews MP, Cheung AM. Well-being in informal caregivers of survivors of acute respiratory distress syndrome. *Crit Care Med*. 2006;34(1):81–86.

90. Cox CE, Docherty SL, Brandon DH, et al. Surviving critical illness: acute respiratory distress syndrome as experienced by patients and their caregivers. *Crit Care Med*. 2009;37(10):2702–2708.

91. Carnevale FA, Alexander E, Davis M, Rennick J, Troini R. Daily living with distress and enrichment: the moral experience of families with ventilator-assisted children at home. *Pediatrics*. 2006;117(1):e48–60.

92. Cuthbertson SJ, Margetts MA, Streat SJ. Bereavement follow-up after critical illness. *Crit Care Med*. 2000;28(4):1196–1201.

93. Choi J, Tate JA, Hoffman LA, et al. Fatigue in family caregivers of adult intensive care unit survivors. *J Pain Symptom Manage*. 2014;48(3):353–363.

94. Titler MG, Cohen MZ, Craft MJ. Impact of adult critical care hospitalization: perceptions of patients, spouses, children, and nurses. *Heart Lung*. 1991;20(2):174–182.

95. Montgomery V, Oliver R, Reisner A, Fallat ME. The effect of severe traumatic brain injury on the family. *J Trauma*. 2002;52(6):1121–1124.

96. Youngblut JM, Singer LT, Boyer C, Wheatley MA, Cohen AR, Grisoni ER. Effects of pediatric head trauma for children, parents, and families. *Crit Care Nurs Clin North Am*. 2000;12(2):227–235.

97. Chien LY, Lo LH, Chen CJ, Chen YC, Chiang CC, Yu Chao YM. Quality of life among primary caregivers of Taiwanese children with brain tumor. *Cancer Nurs*. 2003;26(4):305–311.

98. Pinelli J, Saigal S, Wu Y-WB, et al. Patterns of change in family functioning, resources, coping and parental depression in mothers and fathers of sick newborns over the first year of life. *J Neonatal Nurs*. 2008;14(5):156–165.

99. Kecskes Z, Connors B. Implementation of Australia's 1st webcam in a NICU. *Pediatr Res*. 2011;70(Suppl 5):660.

100. Cox C, Bialoskurski M. Neonatal intensive care: communication and attachment. *Br J Nurs*. 2001;10(10):668–676.

101. Dithole K, Thupayagale-Tshweneagae G, Mgutshini T. Posttraumatic stress disorder among spouses of patients discharged from the intensive care unit after six months. *Issues Ment Health Nurs*. 2013;34(1):30–35.

102. Lemiale V, Kentish-Barnes N, Chaize M, et al. Health-related quality of life in family members of intensive care unit patients. *J Palliat Med*. 2010;13(9):1131–1137.

Note: Page numbers followed by italicized letters indicate *figures*, *tables*, or *boxes*.

activities of daily living, and long-term
    cognitive impairment, 63
acute respiratory distress
    syndrome (ARDS)
  brain atrophy in survivors of, 14–15
  brain imaging following, 14–15
  cognitive impairment in survivors
    of, 11–13
  PTSD phenomena in survivors, 79
acute stress disorder, 120
Acute Stress Disorder Scale (ASDS), 181
age
  and critical illness-related cognitive
    impairment, 57
  as risk factor for long-term cognitive
    impairment, 62
agitation
  in delirium, 32
  as marker of risk for post-ICU
    PTSD, 76–77
Alzheimer's disease, as opposed to
    long-term cognitive impairment,
    58*t*–59*t*
amnesia
  of hospitalization in ICU, 3
  severe illness as cause of, 1–2

analgesia, and preventing and treating
    delirium, 40
anoxia, effects of anoxic brain
    injury, 10–11
antidepressant medications, use in
    critically ill patients, 123
antipsychotic medication, use in treating
    delirium, 40–41
anxiety
  among family members, 197–199
  assessment tools, 119, 131
  and cessation of mechanical ventilation,
    128–129
  effects on sleep, 195
  intervention strategies, 119
  measuring anxiety phenomena, 92–93
  post-ICU therapies for, 8–9, 161–163
  and predisposition for delusional
    memories, 82
  prevalence of in survivors of critical
    illness, 118–119
  as risk factor for post-ICU
    PTSD, 77
  role of delusional memories in,
    6–7, 7*f*, 93
  using ICU diaries to treat, 150–159

assessment
  of anxiety, 119, 131
  of delirium, 33–37, 129
  of health-related behaviors in
    patients, 125
  of medical decision-making capacity,
    109–110
  of PTSD, 120
  and rehabilitation psychology in ICU,
    111t–113t
Atherton, Steve, 2–3
autonomy, stress of reductions in, 75

Beck Depression Inventory-2, 122, 143
benzodiazepines
  discontinuing in treatment of
    delirium, 40
  and post-ICU PTSD, 76–77, 80, 81
bereavement
  physical outcomes of, 201
  social outcomes of, 201–203
Bienvenu, O. Joseph
  "Prevention and Treatment of
    Posttraumatic Stress and Depressive
    Phenomena in Critical Illness
    Survivors," 141–167
  "Psychological Impact of Critical
    Illness," 69–104
body image dissatisfaction, 123
brain atrophy, in survivors of
  ARDS, 14–15
brain imaging, following critical
  illness, 14–15
brain injury
  as cause of cognitive impairment after
    critical illness, 110
  effects of anoxic brain injury, 10–11
  hypoxia as mechanism of, 57, 59
  referrals to specialist, 24–25

Capgras delusion, case history of in
  ICU, 3–4
carbon dioxide, elevated levels of and
  anxiety, 73

cardiopulmonary resuscitation, family
  presence at, 198
caregiving burden
  among family members, 200
  physical outcomes of, 201
  social outcomes of, 201–203
Carlo, Maria E.
  "Critical Illness and Long-Term
    Cognitive Impairment," 47–68
catecholamines
  role in enhancing traumatic memory
    formation, 84
  stress related to high levels of, 74
Center for Epidemiologic
  Studies Depression Scale
  (CES-D), 122
cerebral vascular damage, as mechanism
  of brain injury, 60
cognitive-behavioral therapy
  elements used in rehabilitation
    psychology, 130
  trauma-focused, 163, 184
cognitive bias, among family
  members, 194
cognitive functioning
  assessing before and after critical illness,
    53–54, 55t–56t, 57
  effects of critical illness, 109–114
  goal-management training, 116–117
  and rehabilitation psychology practices,
    111t–112t
  trajectories after critical illness, 50
cognitive impairment
  as brain injury, 110
  epidemiology of, 110, 114
  improving cognitive outcomes, 15–16
  and medical decision-making capacity,
    109–110
  patient perceptions of, 51–52
  in survivors of acute respiratory distress
    syndrome, 11–13
cognitive impairment, long-term
  assessing before and after critical illness,
    53–54, 55t–56t, 57

as compared with delirium and
    Alzheimer's disease, 58t–59t
domains of cognition impaired, 49–50
effects on driving and
    employment, 52–53
epidemiology of, 110, 114
future research on, 63–65
implications of, 62–63
mechanisms of, 57–61
origins and impact of, 47–48
prevalence of, 48–51
as public health issue, 64–65
querying patients regarding
    impacts of, 53
risk factors associated with, 61–62
role of critical illness in
    developing, 48–49
screening to detect, 50–51
cognitive outcomes, improving in
    post-ICU patients, 15–16
cognitive processes, effect of emotions on,
    193–194
cognitive rehabilitation
    case study of, 126–127
    in critical illness survivors, 114–117
    in medical populations, 115–116
communication
    and reducing family-member stress, 198
    stress of limitations in, 74–75
    teach-back method of instruction,
        194–195
    teaching caregiving tasks to family
        members, 200
    while on mechanical ventilation, 129
concentration, addressing issues with,
    126–127
Confusion Assessment Method for ICU
    (CAM-ICU), 33–35, 34t
cortical and subcortical hypoperfusion, as
    mechanism of brain injury, 60
corticosteroids
    and preventing post-ICU PTSD, 80, 145
    and reducing post-ICU PTSD,
        77, 83–85

Colville, Gillian
    "Supporting Pediatric Patients
    and Their Families during and
    after Intensive Care Treatment,"
    169–190
critical illness
    assessing cognitive impairment
        before and after, 53–54,
        55t–56t, 57
    brain imaging following, 14–15
    cognitive effects of, 11–13, 109–114
    cognitive rehabilitation in survivors of,
        114–117
    financial implications of, 202
    functional impact of, 124–125
    psychological effects of, 2–3, 117–123
    speaking on experience of, 27–28
    stress related to, 73–75
    trajectory of recovery from, 117

Davidson, Judy E., 191–209
delirium
    assessing, 33–37
    definition of, 31–32
    effect of on family members, 197–198
    etiology and risk factors, 37–38
    historical observations of, 1–2
    impact of, 33
    as mechanism of brain injury, 110
    and medical decision-making capacity,
        109–110
    occurrence and subtypes of, 32
    in pediatric patients, 173–175, 175b
    predicting and preventing, 38–39
    and rehabilitation of patients on
        mechanical ventilation, 129
    as risk factor for long-term cognitive
        impairment, 61
    as risk factor for post-ICU PTSD,
        76–77, 81–83
    stress experienced with, 74
    treating, 39–41
    vs. long-term cognitive impairment,
        58t–59t

delusions
  and increased sedation, 142–143
  origins of in ICU procedures, 73
  patient accounts of, 20–22, 24, 69–72
  patient demands for explanation of, 5
  predisposing factors for, 82
  reducing impact of delusional
    memories, 7–8
  stress experienced with, 74
  and subsequent anxiety, 6–7, 7f, 93
dementia, ICU hospitalization and other
    risk factors, 54
depression
  among family members, 13–14, 197–199
  and anticipatory grief, 194
  and delusional memories, 82
  etiology and potential consequences
    of, 90f
  interventions for, 122–123
  measuring, 89, 91–92, 122
  phenomenology, 88
  post-ICU depression, growing
    awareness of, 141–142
  post-ICU therapies for, 8–9, 161–163
  prevalence, 88, 121–122
  preventing, 142–148
  rehabilitation programs to treat,
    148–150
  as risk factor for long-term cognitive
    impairment, 62
  risk factors for, 88–89
  using ICU diaries to reduce and treat,
    150–159, 152
  using support groups to treat, 159–161
diaries, ICU
  child's farewell to grandfather, 151f
  history and examples of, 150–159,
    154f, 155b
  as intervention to reduce PTSD, 77, 81,
    150–159
  introducing to patients and family
    members, 153f
  medical glossary for patients and family
    members, 156b–157b
  overall benefits of use, 158–159

patient diaries of post-ICU
    experience, 7–8
  reduced depression and anxiety, 93, 152,
    157–159
  reduced PTSD in family members, 199
  storybook diaries for pediatric patients,
    176b–177b, 178f
driving, and long-term cognitive
    impairment, 52

electroencephalography (EEG), and
    assessing delirium, 37
emotions, effects of among family
    members, 193–194
employment
  and long-term cognitive impairment, 53
  patient account of return to, 24
epidemiology
  of cognitive impairment after critical
    illness, 110, 114
  of post-intensive care syndrome
    (PICS), 171
EuroQol, 122
executive dysfunction, using goal
    management training to address,
    116–117
exercise
  and improving cognitive
    outcomes, 15–16
  and treating depression, 149–150
eyeglasses, and preventing and treating
    delirium, 40
eye movement desensitization and
    reprocessing (EMDR), 162

Facilitated Sensemaking, to improve
    coping among family members, 192
family intensive care unit syndrome
    (FICUS), 192–196
family members
  anxiety, depression, and PTSD among,
    197–199
  caregiving burden among, 200
  child-parent pairs with PTSD
    symptoms, 180f

child's farewell to grandfather in ICU diary, 151*f*

complicated grief among, 200

delirium-specific support for, 197–198

effects of intense emotion among, 193–194

health maintenance among, 191

hope and optimism among, 194

ICU diary glossary for, 156*b*–157*b*

improving quality of life for, 202–203

instituting support groups for, 4–5, 9

intra-family conflict, 195–196

introductory information on ICU diaries, 153*f*

morbidities experienced by, 13–14

of pediatric patients, 172–178

peer-to-peer support in NICU, 199

phases of trauma experience, 171–172

physical outcomes of caregiving and bereavement, 201

post-ICU parental perspectives and adjustments, 179–180

providing structured activities for, 192

role clarification for, 192–193, 195–196

screening for post-PICU parental distress, 181–182

sleep deprivation among, 195

social outcomes of caregiving and bereavement, 201–203

as sources of patient support, 22, 25

structured services to, 170

support for families of children who die, 175, 177, 178, 184

support groups and group meetings for, 159–161

and transition out of ICU, 199

using teach-back method of instruction with, 194–195

family space, in intensive care units, 195

fatigue, types experienced by ICU patients, 129–130

fear

addressing in post-ICU therapy, 8–9

of recurring illness, 71–72, 75

as result of Capgras delusion in ICU, 4

fever, as a marker of risk for delirium, 1–2

financial strain, on family members, 202

Functional Assessment of Cancer Therapy-Cognitive Function (FACT-Cog), 51–52

functional impact of critical illness, 124–125

general hospital ward, and trauma of move from ICU, 20

genetic factors, and risk for long-term cognitive impairment, 62

Gibb, Peter

"The ICU Patient," 17–28

glucose dysregulation, as mechanism of brain injury, 60, 110

goal-management training

addressing issues with concentration and inattention, 127

to enhance cognitive function, 116–117

grief

anticipatory grief among family members, 194

complicated grief, 200

physical outcomes of, 201

social outcomes of, 201–203

Griffiths, Richard, 3

hallucinations

and increased sedation, 142–143

origins of in ICU procedures, 73

patient accounts of, 69–72

patient demands for explanation of, 5

persistent patient memories of, 3

predisposing factors for, 82

stress experienced with, 74

haloperidol, preventing and treating delirium, 39, 41

health-care team, behavior toward family members, 197

health-related behaviors, assessing and addressing, 125

health-related quality of life, 63

hearing aids, preventing and treating delirium, 40

hope, importance of for family members, 194, 195

Hopkins, Ramona O.
  "Critical Illness and Long-Term Cognitive Impairment," 47–68
  "Nurse, Parent, and Researcher," 10–17
  "Rehabilitation Psychology Insights for Treatment of Critical Illness Survivors," 105–139

Hospital Anxiety and Depression Scale (HADS), 91–92, 122, 146

hyperglycemia, as mechanism of brain injury, 60

hypnotherapy, post-ICU, 162

hypoglycemia, as mechanism of brain injury, 60

hypoperfusion, cortical and subcortical, 60

hypotension, 60

hypothalamic-pituitary-adrenal axis, strain placed on, 74

hypoxia
  anxiety related to, 73
  as mechanism of brain injury, 57, 59, 110

ICU diaries
  child's farewell to grandfather, 151f
  and decreased PTSD in family members, 199
  history and examples of, 154f, 155b
  introducing patients and family members to, 153f
  medical glossary for patients and family members, 156b–157b
  overall benefits of use, 158–159
  storybook ICU diaries for pediatric patients, 176b–177b, 178f

ICU memory tool, design and use of, 5–6, 6–7

ICU psychosis
  historical observations of, 2
  patient accounts of, 69–72

ICU Recovery Manual, 148

ICUsteps support group, 9, 25–27, 159–160

Impact of Event Scale-Revised (IES-R), 120, 143

inattention, addressing issues with, 126–127

inflammation
  inflammatory cascade, 74
  as mechanism of brain injury, 60–61, 110
  role of corticosteroids in reducing, 85

instrumental activities of daily living, and long-term cognitive impairment, 63

"Intensive Care: A Guide for Patients and Relatives," booklet, 27

Intensive Care Delirium Screening Checklist (ICDSC), 33–34, 35–37, 36t

intensive care unit (ICU)
  account of becoming a patient, 17–20
  explaining alarms and other alerts to family members, 194
  family space included in, 195
  gathering patient memories of, 5–7, 7f
  neonatal intensive care unit, family interactions in, 193
  patient account of leaving, 20–23
  patient account of move to general ward, 20
  patient return to, 23
  rehabilitation psychology practices in, 111t–113t
  sleep-wake cycle dysregulation in, 118
  speaking on patient experience of, 27–28
  stress related to stay in, 73–75
  transition out of, 199

interventions
  for acute stress disorder, 120
  for anxiety, 119
  benefits of early mobilization, 118
  for posttraumatic stress disorder (PTSD), 121
  and rehabilitation psychology peri ICU, 111t–113t
  for symptoms of posttraumatic stress, 182, 183b–184b

use of cognitive-behavioral therapy,
130–131
intubation, stress related to, 73

Jackson, James C.
"Critical Illness and Long-Term
Cognitive Impairment," 47–68
"Rehabilitation Psychology Insights
for Treatment of Critical Illness
Survivors," 105–139
Jones, Christina
"Prevention and Treatment of
Posttraumatic Stress and Depressive
Phenomena in Critical Illness
Survivors," 141–167
"Psychological Impact of Critical
Illness," 69–104
"The Intensive Care Unit Nurse Turned
Researcher," 1–9
Jutte, Jennifer E.
"Rehabilitation Psychology Insights
for Treatment of Critical Illness
Survivors," 105–139

languages, capacity for in ICU
patients, 19
"learned helplessness," among
family members of ICU
patients, 192
lethargy, in delirium, 32

mechanical ventilation
and caring for children at home, 200
factors to consider in rehabilitation,
128–131
medical decision-making, effects of
delirium on capacity for, 109–110
memories
of childhood trauma, 8–9
gathering patient memories of ICU,
5–7, 7f
of nightmares and hallucinations, 3,
80, 81, 83
in pediatric patients, 174
reducing impact of, 7–8, 161–163

memory
effects of severe illness on, 1–2
lapses of in ICU patients, 18–19
mobilization
benefits of early, 118, 147–148
and preventing delirium, 197–198
and treating delirium, 40
mortality, delirium and increased
rates of, 33
motivational enhancement therapy, 123

narrative exposure therapy, 182,
183b–184b, 185f
Neonatal Individualized Developmental
Care and Assessment Program
(NIDCAP), 193
neonatal intensive care unit (NICU)
family integrity and bonding in,
193, 201
parents and peer-to-peer support
in, 199
Netzer, Giora, 191–209
neuropathology, using brain imaging to
uncover, 14–15
neurotransmitters, pathways implicated in
delirium, 38
nightmares
and increased sedation, 142–143
origins of in ICU procedures, 73
patient accounts of, 69–72
patient demands for explanation of, 5
persistent patient memories of, 3, 19
predisposing factors for, 82
stress experienced with, 74
nurses, role in ICU diaries, 152, 153f
nutrition, positive impact on
depression, 149

occupational therapy, and preventing
delirium, 39
opioid medication
and onset of delirium, 2
as risk factor for post-ICU
PTSD, 76–77
and sleep cycles, 120

optimism, importance of for family
    members, 194

palliative care practice, goals of care
    in, 195
paranoia
    patient account of, 20–22, 24
    patient demands for explanation of, 5
parental distress in PICU
    identifying factors contributing to,
        173–174
    interventions for symptoms of
        posttraumatic stress, 182, 183b–184b
Parental Stressor Scale: PICU (PSS:PICU),
    172–173, 181
Patient Health Questionnaire, 122
patients
    becoming an ICU patient, 17–20
    discharge from ICU, 20–23
    instituting support groups for, 4–5, 9
    integrating patient perspectives into
        research, 65
    marking anniversary of crisis, 25
    perceptions of cognitive impairment,
        51–52, 53
    psychotic experiences in ICU, 69–72
    returning to work, 24
    return visit to ICU, 23
    speaking on experience of critical
        illness, 27–28
    structured post-ICU services to
        families, 169–172
patients, pediatric
    child-parent pairs with post-PICU
        PTSD symptoms, 180f
    delirium in, 173–175
    explaining delirium to, 174–175, 175b
    family support services in acute phase
        of treatment, 172–178
    future directions for post-ICU
        follow-up and care, 185–186
    memories in, 174
    post-ICU parental perspectives and
        adjustments, 179–180

screening for PTSD symptoms in,
    180–182
storybook ICU diaries for,
    176b–177b, 178f
structured support for families of
    children regularly in the PICU, 175,
    177, 180b
Pediatric Medical Traumatic Stress
    (PMTS) model, 171
pediatric patients
    child-parent pairs with post-ICU PTSD
        symptoms, 180f
    delirium in, 173–175
    explaining delirium to, 174–175, 175b
    family support services in acute phase
        of treatment, 172–178
    future directions for post-ICU follow-
        up and care, 185–186
    memories in, 174
    models of care for, 171
    post-ICU parental perspectives and
        adjustments, 179–180
    screening for PTSD symptoms in,
        180–182
    storybook ICU diaries for,
        176b–177b, 178f
    structured services to families, 169–172,
        175, 177, 180b
peer support, and improving cognitive
    outcomes, 16
physical activity, benefits of early
    mobilization, 118
physical function, and rehabilitation
    psychology practices in ICU, 111t
physical rehabilitation
    addressing post-ICU anxiety
        symptoms, 93
    and improving cognitive
        outcomes, 15–16
    and reducing depression, 122–123
physical restraint, and use of sedative
    medication, 83
physical therapy, use in preventing
    delirium, 39

physiotherapy, and treating
    depression, 149
post-intensive care syndrome-family
    (PICS-F), 196–197, 196f
post-intensive care syndrome (PICS)
    addressing risk factors for, 105–106
    characteristics of, 105
    developing uniform epidemiology
        for, 171
    future directions for research and care,
        185–186
    improving cognitive outcomes, 15–16
    introductory studies of, 13–14
    structured services to address, 170
Posttraumatic Adjustment Scale
    (PAS), 181
Posttraumatic Stress Diagnostic Scale, 87
posttraumatic stress disorder (PTSD)
    addressing in post-ICU therapy, 8–9
    among family members, 197–199
    and ARDS, 79
    assessment of, 120
    child-parent pairs with symptoms
        of, 180f
    clinical studies of, 77, 79–88
    and delayed reactions to stress, 181–182
    delirium as risk factor for, 81–83
    effect of post-ICU diaries on, 7–8
    etiology of, 78t
    factors associated with development
        of, 82f
    growing awareness of post-ICU PTSD,
        141–142
    ICU diaries to treat, 150–159
    interventions for treating, 121, 161–163,
        182, 183b–184b
    measuring, 85–88
    phenomenology of, 75
    prevalence of, 76, 120
    preventing post-ICU PTSD, 142–148
    protective factors, 78t
    reducing risk of, 77, 83–85
    rehabilitation programs to treat,
        148–150

risk factors for, 76–77, 78t
role of delusional memories in, 6–7,
    7f, 80, 81
screening for symptoms in pediatric
    patients, 180–182
subsyndromal presentations of
    symptoms, 182
in survivors of critical illness, 79–81
using support groups to treat, 159–161
Post-Traumatic Stress Syndrome
    10-Questions Inventory, 85–88,
    120, 144
problem-solving therapy, for reducing
    depressive symptoms, 123
prognosis, reaction of family members
    to, 194
Program of Enhanced Physiotherapy &
    Structured Exercise (PEPSE), 149
psychiatric morbidity post-ICU, studies
    examining, 93–95
psychological effects of critical illness,
    117–123
psychological functioning, and rehabilitation
    psychology practices peri ICU, 112t
psychological impact of critical illness
    anxiety, 92–93
    depression, 88–89, 89, 90f, 91–92
    historical observations of, 2–3
    posttraumatic stress disorder, 78f, 82f
    posttraumatic stress disorder, studies
        regarding, 77–88
    posttraumatic stress phenomena, 75–77
    psychotic experiences, patient
        descriptions of, 69–72
    reducing impact of delusional
        memories, 7–8
    significance of stress in, 73–75
    studies examining, 93–95
psychological rehabilitation, case study of,
    128–131
psychological support, intra-ICU, 145–147
psychosis
    historical observations of, 2
    patient accounts of episodes in ICU, 69–72

quality of life
  and functional impact of critical
    illness, 124
  improving for family members,
    202–203
  and rehabilitation psychology
    assessment and intervention peri
    ICU, 113t

RACHEL research group, 7, 8, 82–83
Reboul-Lachaux, J., 3–4
recovery from critical illness, trajectory
  of, 117
rehabilitation
  and improving cognitive
    outcomes, 15–16
  to treat posttraumatic stress and
    depression, 148–150
rehabilitation psychology
  assessing and treating health-related
    behaviors, 125
  assessment and intervention in the ICU,
    111t–113t
  case study of cognitive rehabilitation,
    126–127
  case study of psychological
    rehabilitation, 128–131
  cognitive rehabilitation in critical illness
    survivors, 114–117
  cognitive rehabilitation in medical
    populations, 115–116
  considerations across continuum of
    care, 108f
  elements of cognitive-behavioral
    therapy used in, 130
  focus of, 106
  goal-management training to enhance
    cognitive function, 116–117
  relevance to treatment of critical illness
    survivors, 106–107, 109
  role of psychologist in ICU, 105–106,
    131–132
  vocational assessment, 124–125
  working with patients on mechanical
    ventilation, 128–131

reorientation, sensory, and treating
  delirium, 40
respiratory insufficiency, anxiety
  related to, 73
Richmond Agitation-Sedation Scale, 34
rivastigmine, and treating delirium, 41
role strain
  assessing families for, 195–196
  and caregiving, 201
Rood, Paul
  "Delirium in Critically Ill
    Patients," 31–45

Screening Tool for Early Predictors of
  PTSD, 181
sedation, and post-ICU PTSD, 79,
  142–144
Sedation-Agitation Scale, 34
sedative medication
  minimizing in delirium prevention, 39
  and onset of delirium, 2
  use in patients with preexisting
    psychological difficulties, 82
  use with physical restraints, 83
sensory reorientation, and treating
  delirium, 40
sepsis and septic shock
  administration of corticosteroids in, 145
  brain injury associated with, 60, 61
sleep
  effect of opioid medication on, 120
  role in preventing delirium, 39, 40
  sleep deprivation among family
    members, 195
  sleep-wake cycle dysregulation in
    ICU, 118
social support, and improving outcomes,
  125–126
Society of Critical Care Medicine, 16,
  170, 196
State Anxiety Inventory, 143
stress
  acute stress disorder, 120
  related to critical illness and intensive
    care, 73–75

Structured Clinical Interview for DSM-IV
  (SCID-IV), 85–86
substance use and abuse, and rehabilitation psychology assessment and
  intervention, 113t, 125
suicide, patient account of brief
  attempt, 23
support groups, patient and family
  disease-specific support groups, 199
  ICUsteps group, 9, 25–27
  instituting, 4–5, 9
  treating depression and PTSD, 159–161
support services
  for families of pediatric patients in acute
    phase of treatment, 172–178
  long-term support for families of
    pediatric patients, 178–186
  structured post-ICU services to families,
    169–172

teach-back method of instruction,
  194–195

therapy
  addressing post-ICU issues in, 8–9
  cognitive-behavioral therapy used in
    rehabilitation, 130
  post-ICU therapies, 161–163
THRIVE initiative, Society of Critical Care
  Medicine, 16
time, changes in awareness of, 20, 23
trauma
  ICU and recall of childhood trauma, 8–9
  phases of trauma experience for
    families, 171–172

Van Den Boogaard, Mark
  "Delirium in Critically Ill
    Patients," 31–45
vocational difficulties, 124–125

work
  patient account of return to, 24
  return to work by family members, 202
  workplace accommodations, 124–125